A Colour Atlas of
Removable Partial Dentures

A Colour Atlas of

Removable Partial Dentures

John C. Davenport
PhD, BDS, FDSRCS.
Senior Lecturer in Dental Prosthetics, University of Birmingham.
Consultant Dental Surgeon, Central Birmingham Health Authority.
External Examiner, University of Glasgow.

Robin M. Basker
DDS, MGDSRCS, LDSRCS.
Professor of Dental Prosthetics, University of Leeds.
Consultant in Restorative Dentistry, Leeds Western Health Authority.
External Examiner, Universities of London, Manchester and Newcastle,
Royal College of Surgeons of England, formerly External Examiner,
Universities of Birmingham, Bristol, Dundee, Sheffield and Wales.

John R. Heath
PhD, BDS, FDSRCS.
Senior Lecturer in Prosthetic Dentistry, University of Manchester.
Consultant in Restorative Dentistry, Central Manchester Health Authority.
Examiner, Royal College of Surgeons of Edinburgh.

James P. Ralph
DDS, FDSRCS, HDD, RCPS.
Consultant in Restorative Dentistry, Leeds Western Health Authority.
Senior Clinical Lecturer, University of Leeds.
Examiner, Royal College of Physicians and Surgeons of Glasgow.

Wolfe Medical Publications Ltd

Copyright © J. C. Davenport, R. M. Basker, J. R. Heath
and J. P. Ralph, 1988
Published by Wolfe Medical Publications Ltd, 1988
Printed by W. S. Cowell Ltd, Ipswich, England
ISBN 0 7234 1035 6

This book is one of the titles in the series of Wolfe Medical
Atlases, a series which brings together probably the world's
largest systematic published collection of diagnostic colour
photographs.
    For a full list of Atlases in the series, plus forthcoming
titles and details of our surgical, dental and veterinary
Atlases, please write to
Wolfe Medical Publications Ltd, 2–16 Torrington Place,
London WC1E 7LT.

Contents

Acknowledgements

The foundations of any atlas are the illustrations and we are greatly indebted to Miss A. Durbin, Department of Medical Illustration, Leeds University, and to Miss S. Davenport for their expert help with the preparation of the diagrams.

We should also like to express our gratitude to Mr A. J. Robertson, Mr P. Parkinson and Mr D. A. Hawkridge of Leeds Dental School and to Mr M. Sharland of Birmingham Dental School for undertaking much of the photography; to Mr F. G. Beanland, Mr B. S. Dransfield and Mr R. Ruddy, Leeds, and Mr W. B. Hullah and Mr D. Spence, Birmingham, for the technical work; to those colleagues, Dr A. Harrison, Dr M. J. Kowolik, Dr F. J. Kratochvil, Mr S. L. Pearson, Miss K. Powell and Dr R. T. Walker, who allowed us to include their photographs; and to Dr H. J. Wilson and Professor W. R. E. Laird for helpful advice.

Preface

Much clinical research over the last three decades has drawn attention to the tissue damage that can occur as a result of removable partial dentures being worn. In the last ten years or so the influence of removable partial dentures on plaque formation has been stressed. There is thus some evidence to support the layman's comment that 'A partial denture is a device for losing one's teeth slowly, painfully and expensively'.

Fortunately, results from other clinical studies redress the balance, indicating that treatment will be successful and that oral health can be maintained, provided that a team approach is adopted – the team comprising the clinician, the dental technician and the patient. The clinician's responsibilities include preparing the patient to accept the partial dentures, designing the dentures carefully so that the risk of damage is reduced to a minimum, undertaking the clinical work to the highest possible standard and communicating with the dental technician so that the details of design are not absent by default. The dental technician's responsibility is to ensure that the dentures are constructed accurately and that the principles of good design are followed through. All this effort is worthless unless the patient appreciates the importance of oral hygiene and prevention of disease and is prepared to put considerable effort into maintaining the mouth and the dentures.

This Atlas attempts to present in pictures and words the principles which govern successful treatment throughout the stages of patient evaluation, denture design, preparation of the mouth and construction of the dentures. We have purposely concentrated on clasp-retained partial dentures as there are other texts which deal with fixed restorations and precision attachments.

Rather than include an exhaustive list of references we have leant heavily on the book *Restoration of the partially dentate mouth,* edited by Bates, Neill and Preiskel, which is a record of a very successful international symposium held in London in 1982. Twelve workshops were held and the reports of these workshops brought together the literature. We feel that this volume provides a useful source of reference for those readers who wish to delve further into that literature.

We have decided to use the FDI two-digit system of tooth notation as it is now becoming more widely accepted throughout the world, probably due to the increasing use of computers. A word of explanation serves as a guide to those readers who have not used it before. The four quadrants of the mouth are denoted by the first digit of each pair of numbers, namely $\frac{1\,/\,2}{4\,/\,3}$. The second digit refers to the tooth, for example:

$$\underline{18\ \ 17\ \ 16\ \ 15\ \ 14\ \ 13\ \ 12\ \ 11\ \ /}$$

Thus, $\underline{4/}$ (upper right first premolar) is 14.

No book can be all-embracing. There is, after all, no real substitute for experience gained by treating patients. We hope, however, that this Atlas will serve as a useful guide to clinical work and that it will encourage the team approach to the care of partially edentulous patients.

J.C.D.
R.M.B.
J.R.H.
J.P.R.

Dedication

We dedicate this book to our wives who have cheerfully endured numerous weekends disrupted by authors' meetings and who have encouraged us throughout the project, showing the greatest of patience and understanding.

Part 1
Patient assessment

The first chapter discusses the advantages and disadvantages that accrue from fitting a partial denture. There follows a reminder of the relevant aspects of intra-oral anatomy together with jaw and occlusal relationships (Chapters 2 and 3).

By applying this knowledge to the clinical stages of history and examination of the patient, information is obtained to develop a diagnosis and provisional treatment plan (Chapter 4). However, before the treatment plan can be finalised, it is necessary to obtain further information by examining study casts obtained from preliminary impressions of the patient's mouth (Chapter 5). These casts may need to be mounted on an articulator (Chapter 6).

1 The partial denture equation

The title of this opening chapter of the Atlas requires immediate explanation. The term 'equation' refers to the balance which must be struck between the good and the bad which can arise from partial dentures. In this chapter we explore the benefits conferred on the patient by a partial denture and, at the same time, highlight the possible risks of tissue damage by such a denture. Ultimately, the decision on whether or not to provide a partial denture will be influenced by a consideration of this equation and also by the level of patient motivation.

Benefits of partial dentures

Appearance

1 The restoration of the missing 12, 11 and 21 is of undeniable benefit to this patient, an 18-year-old girl, and the motivation to wear the denture is understandably strong. Particular attention has been paid to the appearance of the denture by the careful choice of artificial teeth and design of the flange. A natural appearance has been created by using a 'veined' acrylic, by reproducing the pre-extraction form of alveolar ridge and by making the distal margin of the flange thin and irregular, thus masking the transition from flange to adjacent mucosa.

1

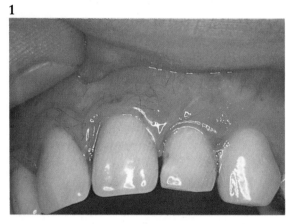

2a

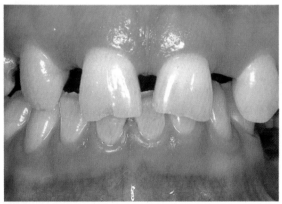

2b

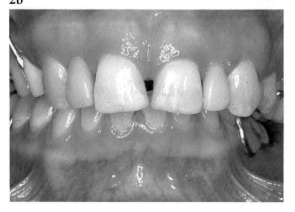

2a and **2b** Not only may a partial denture help to restore appearance but it may actually improve it.
(a)   This patient's upper lateral incisors had never developed and she was concerned about the spacing of the anterior teeth.
(b)   The combination of orthodontic movement of the central incisors and the provision of partial dentures improved the appearance.

3 If an incisor is not replaced soon after extraction, successful treatment at a later date may be compromised. Here, the adjacent teeth have drifted into the unrestored 21 space. The reduced space does not allow an artificial tooth of a realistic size to be used on a denture. If a reasonable aesthetic result is to be obtained the space must be re-established by orthodontic treatment.

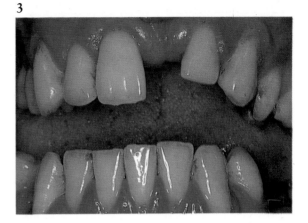

Speech

4 The loss of upper anterior teeth may prevent the clear reproduction of certain sounds, particularly the 'F' and 'V' which are made by the lower lip contacting the edges of the upper incisors. The replacement of missing upper anterior teeth will make a significant contribution to the quality of speech.

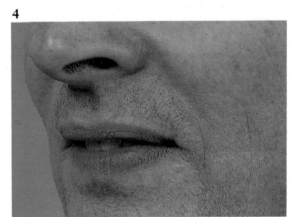

Mastication

5 With modern foods and methods of preparation it is unlikely that a patient will suffer from malnutrition even though a large number of teeth are missing. However, the gaps which arise through the loss of posterior teeth reduce the efficiency of mastication by allowing the bolus of food to slip into the edentulous areas and thus escape the crushing and shearing action of the remaining teeth. A well-fitting denture will prevent this escape of the bolus and thus contribute to masticatory efficiency.

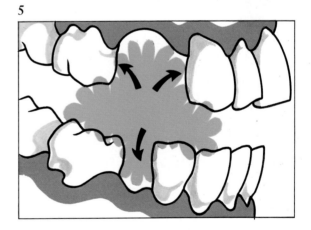

Maintaining the health of the masticatory system

The provision of a partial denture can make a positive contribution to oral health by preventing, or minimising, the undesirable consequences of tooth loss as described in the following paragraphs.

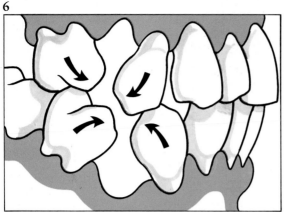

Preventing undesirable tooth movement

6 When teeth are lost from a dental arch the teeth adjacent to the edentulous space may tilt and move into that space. The drift of a tooth into an unrestored space opens up a further space between it and its immediate neighbour. The opportunity of food impaction and plaque formation in the interdental space is increased, encouraging inflammation of the periodontal tissues and decalcification of the proximal surfaces of the teeth. Inevitably, the longer the space remains unrestored the greater the chance of tooth movement. When teeth are lost from an opposing arch overeruption is likely to occur with similar deleterious effects on oral health.

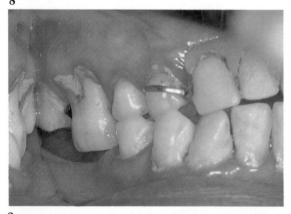

7 The long-term absence of antagonists has resulted in overeruption of upper and lower teeth. The teeth are virtually contacting the opposing edentulous ridges creating major problems if partial dentures have to be provided.

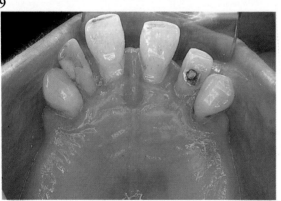

8 In this example, 16 has overerupted to such an extent that it has lost most of its bony support. Extraction of the tooth is inevitable.

Improved distribution of occlusal load

9 The loss of a large number of teeth puts an increasing functional burden on the remainder. In the first example there is existing periodontal disease. The increased functional load has hastened the destruction of the periodontal attachments of the upper anterior teeth which have become increasingly mobile and have drifted labially.

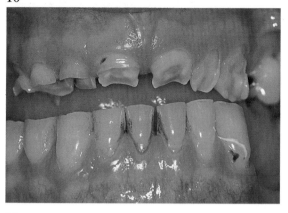

10   If the periodontal attachments of the remaining teeth are healthy, the increased load may result in excessive tooth wear or may cause damage to existing restorations. The restoration of gross loss of tooth substance, as in this example, is likely to involve complex and prolonged treatment.

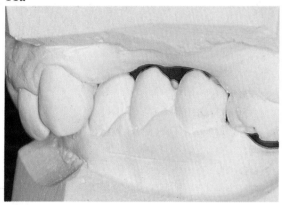

11a and **11b**   Overeruption of a tooth may place it in such a position that it bears the brunt of the occlusal load on initial contact or in excursive movements of the mandible and therefore it may well be subjected to excessive force. In addition, where overeruption of a tooth has created an occlusal interference (*), the patient may modify the habitual movement patterns of the mandible in order to avoid the interfering contact. Although such a modification may reduce the force applied to the tooth, the changed pattern in activity of the mandibular musculature may produce muscular dysfunction.

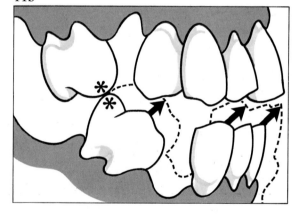

From the foregoing examples it will be appreciated that if tooth loss is restored in sufficient time to prevent tooth movement, or to avoid excessive stress being placed on the remaining structures, the subsequent health of the oral tissues can benefit considerably. However, the point should be made that severe damage is not an inevitable consequence of tooth loss. The implications of this statement will become more apparent later in this section when the damaging effects of the dentures themselves are described.

Preparation for complete dentures

Most of this book is devoted to the treatment of patients who are expected to retain their remaining natural teeth for a considerable number of years, thus allowing the partial denture to be regarded as a long-term restoration. But we should remember those patients whose remaining teeth carry a relatively poor prognosis and for whom, in due course, complete dentures are inevitable. If simple acrylic partial dentures are provided, the patient is able to serve a prosthetic 'apprenticeship' with appliances which receive some stability from the few remaining teeth. In the fullness of time the dentures become more extensive as further teeth are extracted and the patient is gradually eased into the totally artificial dentition. This form of transitional treatment can be of considerable benefit, especially for the elderly patient.

12

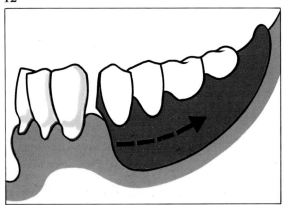

12 The location of the remaining teeth plays an important part in the success of such a transitional denture. It is common for the six lower anterior teeth to be the last remaining teeth in the lower jaw. A denture restoring the posterior teeth is frequently not worn by the patient for the following reasons: first, the denture may be unstable because there is little resistance to its displacement in a posterior direction; second, there is very little motivation to wear the denture as the anterior teeth are still present.

13

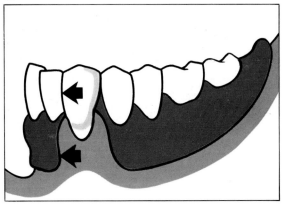

13 If, instead of extracting all the teeth, the canines are retained, the denture will be more stable. As the denture replaces anterior teeth it is very much more likely to be worn and thus the patient is likely to gain greater benefit from the transitional denture.

14   It should be remembered that the transitional partial denture is being placed in a mouth where existing dental disease is only poorly controlled. As will be seen in the next section, the very presence of a denture aggravates the situation. If the mouth is not inspected regularly to identify treatment needs as they arise, there is the likelihood of acceleration of tissue damage which may prejudice the eventual complete denture foundation.

In this case the inflammation and hyperplasia of the palatal mucosa was so severe that surgery had to be performed before further prosthetic treatment could be undertaken.

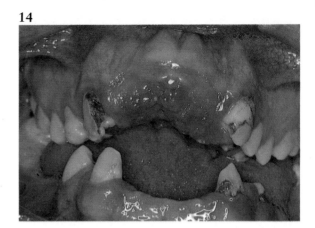

14

Causes of damage related to the wearing of partial dentures

Harmful effects can arise from the plaque which is likely to accumulate around any partial denture, from direct trauma by individual components of the denture, from excessive functional forces which will be transmitted by an ill-designed prosthesis and from errors in the occlusion. The causes and sequelae, summarised in the accompanying table, will now be considered in greater detail.

Summary of damage that may result from wearing a partial denture

Causes	Teeth	Periodontal tissues	Edentulous areas	Muscles of mastication
Plaque accumulation	Decalcification and caries	Inflammation of gingival tissues. Progression to underlying structures	Inflammation of mucous membrane	
Direct trauma from components	Abrasion and fracture of restorations	Inflammation of gingival tissues. Progression to underlying structures	Localised inflammation of mucous membrane. Denture-induced hyperplasia	
Transmission of excessive functional forces		a) Tooth mobility b) Aggravation of existing periodontal disease	Inflammation of mucous membrane. Resorption of bone	
Occlusal error		a) Tooth mobility b) Aggravation of existing periodontal disease	Inflammation of mucous membrane. Resorption of bone	Muscle dysfunction

Increased plaque accumulation

During the last few years a considerable amount of research effort has been directed towards an understanding of the relationship between plaque accumulation and the wearing of partial dentures. It is possible that the presence of a denture influences the quality of the plaque; it certainly affects the quantity. Not only does more plaque accumulate around the teeth in the jaw in which the denture is placed, but more is found around the teeth in the opposing jaw unless the patient is instructed in meticulous oral hygiene procedures.

15a

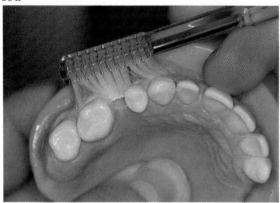

15b

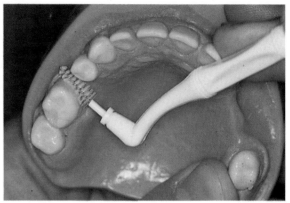

15a and **15b**   The areas which collect most plaque are the proximal surfaces of abutment teeth adjacent to the saddle. (**a**) These surfaces are difficult to clean when using a conventional tooth brush. (**b**) An interdental brush is more effective.

16a

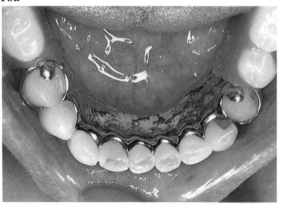

16b

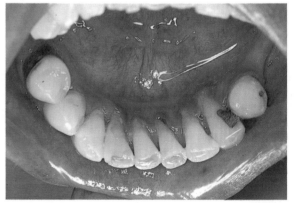

16a and **16b**   The design of the denture may have a significant effect on plaque accumulation. For example, it has been shown that more plaque collects under a lingual plate than under a lingual bar. (**a**) The lingual plate is well supported on the natural teeth and fits well against tooth surfaces. (**b**) However, gingival inflammation has been caused by the increased accumulation of plaque.

17 If the plaque is allowed to persist, the inflammatory process will progress to the deeper tissues, resulting in a chronic periodontitis. The periodontal attachment is progressively destroyed, a periodontal pocket develops and the investing alveolar bone is lost.

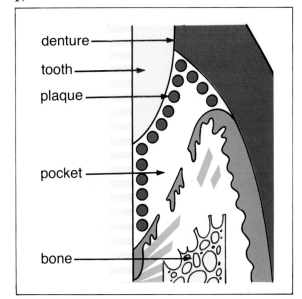

18 Unless the increased accumulation of plaque is removed, root caries is highly likely, a problem which will increase as more patients continue to wear partial dentures into old age.

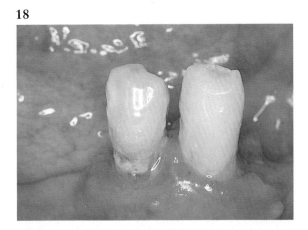

19 If plaque is allowed to collect between the denture and the denture-bearing mucosa, a generalised inflammation, termed denture stomatitis, will be produced. In this case the extent of the denture stomatitis is demarcated precisely by the palatal shape of the denture. This condition is discussed more fully in Chapter 16.

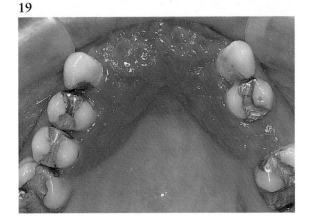

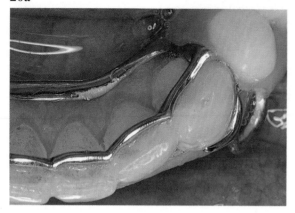

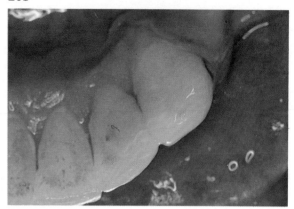

Direct trauma from components

20a and **20b** The oral mucosa is vulnerable to direct trauma from components of dentures. (**a**) In this instance the lingual bar has been positioned too close to the gingival margin. The continuous clasp offers only limited tooth support for the denture. (**b**) The denture has sunk into the tissues, stripping away the gingival tissues on the distal and lingual aspects of 33.

There is no evidence for the contention that a clasp arm will wear the enamel surface to a degree which is significant clinically. However, the movement of a clasp arm may wear the surface of restorative materials, especially composites and dental amalgams.

Transmission of excessive force

Functional forces are transmitted by a partial denture to the tissues with which it is in contact. If a denture is supported primarily by the natural teeth most of the forces will be transmitted to the alveolar bone through the fibres of the peridontal ligament. Bearing in mind the orientation of most of these fibres, it will be appreciated that the forces are tensile in nature and are dissipated over a relatively large area. A very different state of affairs exists when a denture is supported only by the mucosa and bone. Here the forces, largely compressive in nature, are transmitted over a restricted area.

21a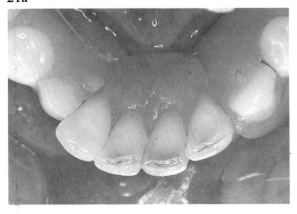

21b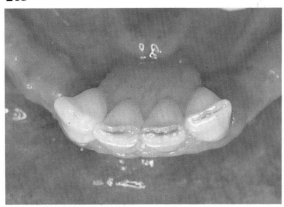

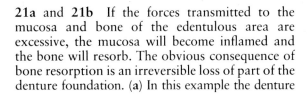

21a and **21b** If the forces transmitted to the mucosa and bone of the edentulous area are excessive, the mucosa will become inflamed and the bone will resorb. The obvious consequence of bone resorption is an irreversible loss of part of the denture foundation. (a) In this example the denture is supported only on the tissues of the edentulous area. It has caused resorption of the bone to such an extent that the lingual bar connector has been pushed down towards the floor of the mouth. (b) The amount of bone which has been destroyed is apparent when the denture is removed.

22 If the design of the denture is such that it transmits excessive force to a tooth there is every likelihood that the tooth will become mobile.

In this example the incorrectly designed cingulum rest (1) transmits a horizontal force to the canine tooth. Such horizontal forces are especially damaging to the periodontal tissues. The incisal rest (2) transmits a more favourable vertical load.

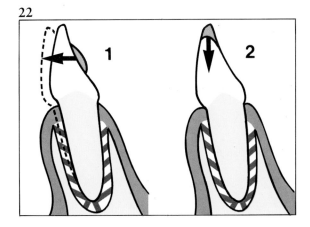

Where periodontal changes are restricted to the marginal gingivae, elimination of excessive force will usually allow the periodontal attachment to return to a normal healthy state. Where the supporting structures have been affected by periodontal disease there is unlikely to be complete resolution.

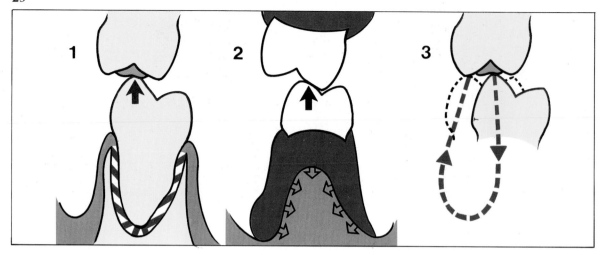

Occlusal error

23 If the occlusal surface of the partial denture is not designed correctly, normal jaw closure may be prevented by a premature occlusal contact. There are three possible sequelae: (1) If the premature contact is on a natural tooth, damage to the tooth or its periodontal ligament will occur. (2) If the saddle bears the brunt of the force of closure, there will be localised mucosal inflammation and resorp- tion of the underlying bone. (3) If the patient attempts to steer the mandible around the pre- mature contact until a more comfortable occlusal position is found, this abnormal closing pattern throws increased demands on certain muscles of mastication, which may result in the patient complaining of facial pain.

Balancing the partial denture equation

Most longitudinal studies have shown quite clearly that the types of damage itemised in the last section are commonly found amongst wearers of partial dentures. Of considerable concern are reports that many patients expressed satisfaction with their dentures in spite of the fact that dental health had deter- iorated markedly. Perhaps this finding is not altogether surprising when we remember the insidious nature of the progression of caries and periodontal disease.

With greater understanding of the relation- ship between plaque and dental disease and of the importance of plaque control, reports have emerged whose findings make for more encouraging reading. There is now firm evidence that the wearing of partial dentures is compatible with continued oral health. This satisfactory outcome depends upon a three- man effort, that of the dentist, that of the dental technician and that of the patient.

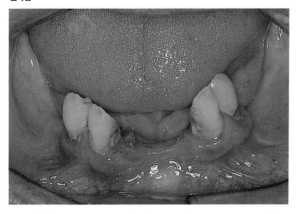

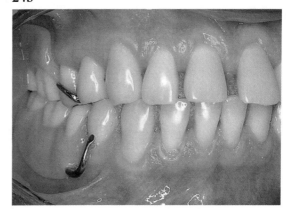

Effort of the dentist

24a and **24b** The primary responsibility of the dentist is to ensure that the remaining teeth and supporting tissues are restored to a healthy state and that the patient is effectively motivated and instructed in how to maintain this state. (**a**) This mouth is not in a fit state to receive a partial denture. There is chronic periodontal disease and accumulation of plaque. (**b**) This patient has responded well to instruction in oral hygiene and the periodontal tissues are healthy. The dangers of wearing the partial dentures are thus minimised.

The second area of responsibility of the dentist is in relation to the construction of the denture. Accuracy of the clinical procedures must, of course, be ensured. In addition, the dentist should produce a design based on criteria which have been shown to promote continued oral health:

Effective support
Clearance of gingival margins
Simplicity
Rigid connector

These criteria will be considered in greater detail in Part 2.

Effort of the technician

25 The technician's effort is directed towards the careful translation of the prescribed denture design into the denture itself and accurate construction and positioning of the denture components. In this instance the inaccurate fit will encourage plaque formation with consequent periodontal disease and caries, thus introducing an unnecessary and avoidable risk to oral health.

25

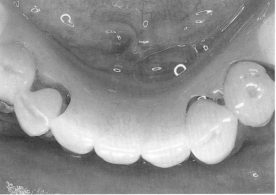

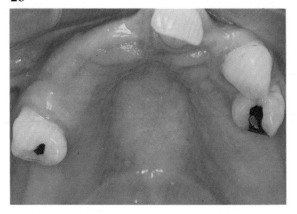

Effort of the patient

26 It is probably true to say that a patient who maintains immaculate plaque control and has a good tissue resistance, or 'host response', can be provided with a less than satisfactory design of denture and still maintain good oral health – such is the importance of the patient's contribution to the partial denture equation. This patient has worn an upper partial denture for many years. The gingival tissues are healthy and the teeth are well supported by bone; all this in spite of the fact that there is little opportunity to provide tooth support.

For every patient, when a denture is contemplated, it is the dentist's responsibility to assess the advantages and disadvantages for that particular mouth; the level of disadvantage is influenced primarily by the level of the patient's dental awareness and plaque control. When the balance of the equation is disturbed towards the side of disadvantage it may well be in the patient's best interest that a denture is not prescribed. Of course, where a denture is required to replace an anterior tooth or teeth, the demand from the patient will usually be overwhelming even if the level of plaque control is less than satisfactory.

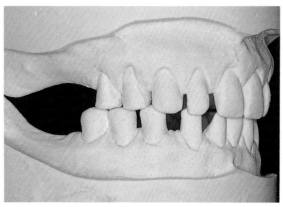

27a

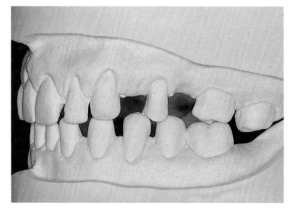

27b

27a and **27b** In this mouth the reasons for providing dentures are not overwhelming. There are sufficient teeth at the front of the mouth to satisfy the demands of appearance and speech. There are certainly enough teeth to allow a varied diet to be eaten. Most of the teeth have antagonists in the opposing arch.

If the mouth is well cared for and the patient desires dentures, the partial denture equation is favourably balanced. However, if plaque control is suspect, there is a strong argument for advising against dentures, at least for a few months until the long-term response to oral hygiene advice is ascertained.

2 Anatomy of the denture-bearing areas

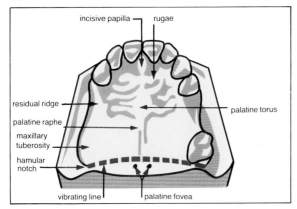

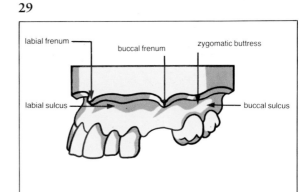

28 and **29**   Surface anatomy of the maxilla.

30   **Incisive papilla.** This soft pad of tissue overlies the incisive canal through which pass the nerves and vessels supplying the anterior part of the palatal mucosa. The labial surfaces of the natural central incisors lie approximately 1 cm anterior to the centre of the papilla, a relationship which should be borne in mind when positioning the artificial replacements.

30

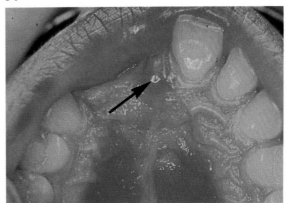

31   **Rugae.** Irregular transverse mucosal ridges occurring in the anterior part of the hard palate. This is an area of fine tactile discrimination and partial dentures should therefore be designed to leave as much of this area uncovered as possible. From this point of view, the anterior border of the denture shown here is preferable to the border indicated by the dotted line.

31

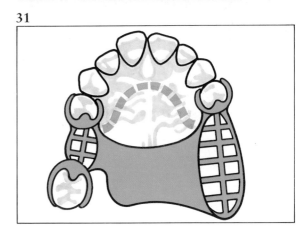

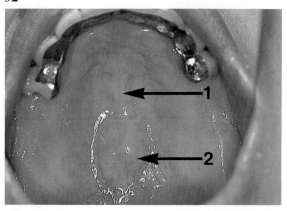

32 (1) **Palatine raphe.** A mucosal ridge lying sagittally in the midline of the palate.

(2) **Palatine torus.** A developmental bony prominence sometimes seen in the centre of the palate. This structure is often covered by relatively incompressible mucoperiosteum. A mucosally supported denture may need to be relieved over the torus to prevent the denture rocking and flexing about the midline.

33

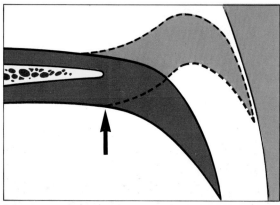

33 **Vibrating line.** The junction between the movable mucosa of the soft palate and the static mucosa of the hard palate. If a decision has been taken to cover a large area of palate with the partial denture connector, the posterior border of the connector should be positioned on the compressible tissue just anterior to the vibrating line.

34

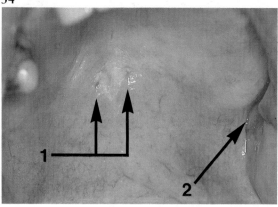

34 (1) **Palatine fovea.** The orifices of common collecting ducts of minor palatine salivary glands which are often to be found close to the vibrating line.

(2) **Hamular notch.** A mucosal depression posterior to the maxillary tuberosity. The notch overlies the gap between the pterygoid hamulus and the maxillary tuberosity and marks the posterior limit of extension of an upper saddle where there is no distal abutment tooth.

35

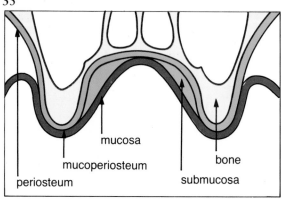

mucosa

mucoperiosteum

bone

periosteum

submucosa

35 **Palatine submucosa.** Variation in thickness of the submucosa influences the compressibility of the denture-bearing surface and consequently the degree of mucosal support offered to a partial denture.

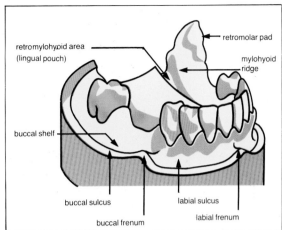

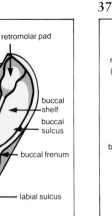

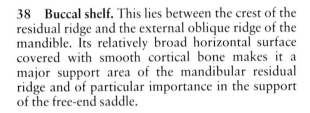

36 and 37   Surface anatomy of the mandible.

38   Buccal shelf. This lies between the crest of the residual ridge and the external oblique ridge of the mandible. Its relatively broad horizontal surface covered with smooth cortical bone makes it a major support area of the mandibular residual ridge and of particular importance in the support of the free-end saddle.

38

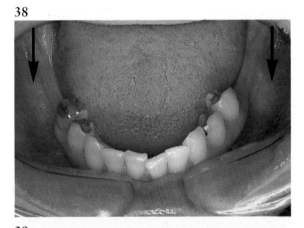

39   Retromolar pad. The anterior part of this pad is usually firm and fibrous and forms an important part of the denture-bearing area. It offers support to the denture and helps to resist posterior displacement. The posterior part is mobile and falls outside the denture-bearing area.

  In the absence of upper and lower posterior teeth, a point halfway up the retromolar pad may be used to indicate the level of the occlusal plane posteriorly.

39

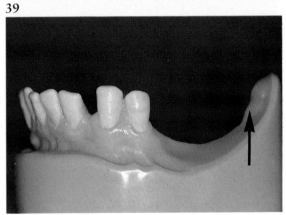

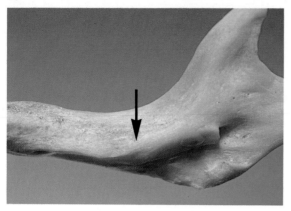

40 Mylohyoid ridge. The bony ridge to which the mylohyoid muscle is attached.

As resorption of the residual ridge proceeds, the prominence of the mylohyoid ridge tends to increase, predisposing to mucosal soreness beneath the denture in this area.

41

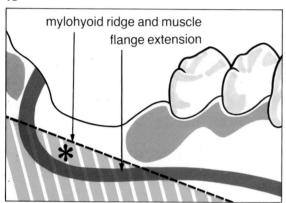

mylohyoid ridge and muscle
flange extension

41 Retromylohyoid area * (lingual pouch). The part of the lingual sulcus lying behind the mylohyoid ridge posteriorly. Whenever the functional movements of the sulcus permit, the lingual flange of a free-end saddle should be extended into this area to provide optimum stability.

42

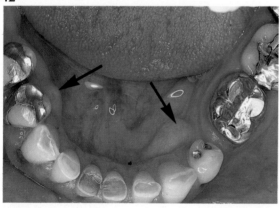

42 Mandibular tori. Developmental bony swellings occasionally seen lingually in the premolar region. They are bilateral, sometimes multiple and usually symmetrical. Mandibular tori may prevent optimum positioning of a lingual major connector and if so may need to be removed surgically.

43

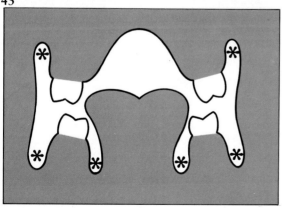

43 Sulcus. The mucosal trough * lying between the ridge on the one hand and the cheeks, lips or tongue on the other. An accurate impression of the functional depth and width of the sulci is necessary because, in the majority of cases, the denture flanges will need to fill the dimensions of the sulci so recorded. It is particularly important to obtain an accurate recording of the form of the lingual sulcus because this will determine the design and positioning of lingual connectors.

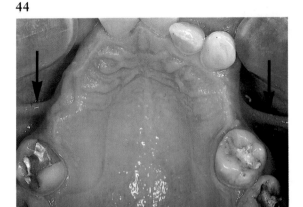

44 Frenum. A fold of mucous membrane which crosses the sulcus and which contains a fibrous submucosa but no muscle fibres. Frena occur buccally in the premolar regions and also in the midline. They require sufficient clearance by the border of a denture to allow their unimpeded movement in function.

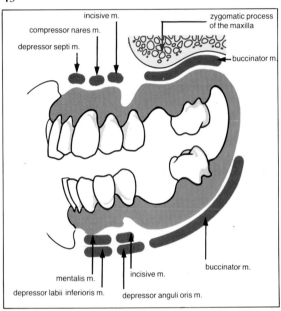

45 Anatomy of the buccal sulci related to the borders of the upper and lower dentures.

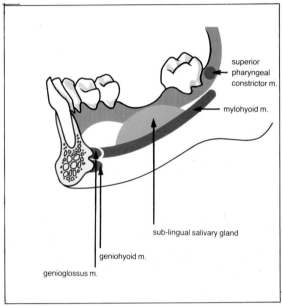

46 Anatomy of the lingual sulci related to the border of the lower denture.

47 Modiolus. This is a decussation of muscle fibres near the angle of the lips. The modiolus can fix the corner of the mouth in any position required for function and during mastication it closes the buccal sulci to prevent escape of the bolus of food.

B   buccinator m.
DAO depressor anguli oris m.
II   incisivus inferior m.
IS   incisivus superior m.
LAO levator anguli oris m.
OO   orbicularis oris m.
ZM   zygomaticus major m.

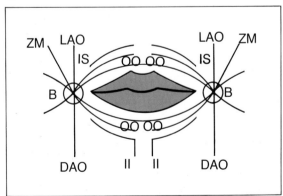

So far in this chapter we have concentrated on the static relationship of oral structures to partial dentures. However, the dynamic relationships also need to be considered.

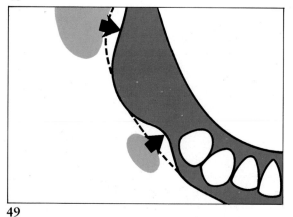

48 On clenching the teeth the anterior border of the masseter muscle bulges into the distobuccal sulcus area. If the flange of a denture is over-extended in this area the resulting pressure may lead to soreness and displacement of the denture.

Failure to contour the buccal flange of a lower denture in the premolar region to accommodate the activity of the modiolus is likely to result in displacement of the denture.

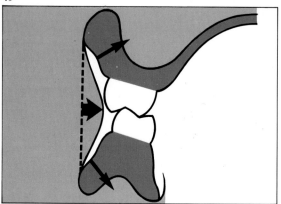

49 Contraction of the buccinator muscle raises a soft-tissue band at about the level of the occlusal plane. The polished surface of a buccal flange should be shaped so that the pressure falling on it from this buccinator activity will have a component of force which is directed towards the ridge and which will therefore help to retain, rather than dislodge, the denture.

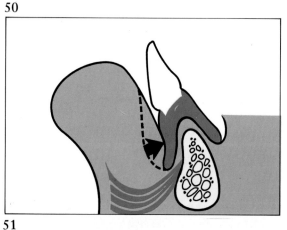

50 Contraction of the mentalis muscle raises the soft tissues of the chin, thus reducing the depth and width of the labial sulcus. If there has been marked resorption of the underlying bone, this muscle can exert considerable pressure on the labial flange of a partial denture, resulting in posterior and upward displacement.

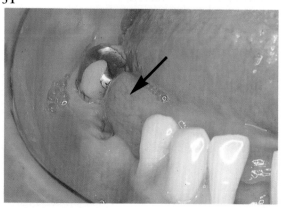

51 When the tongue is elevated, the sublingual folds are raised and may greatly reduce the depth and width of the lingual sulcus. This phenomenon is most marked when advanced resorption of the ridge has occurred.

52 When the mandible is moved laterally, the coronoid process on the non-working side (the side from which the mandible is moving) comes into close relationship to the buccal aspect of the maxillary tuberosity. The buccal sulcus in this region is thus reduced in width, limiting the space available for a buccal flange.

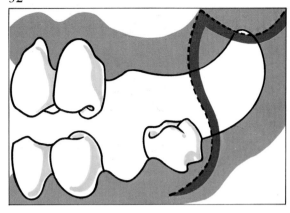

3 Jaw relationships

Jaw relationships may be considered from an anatomical and from a functional viewpoint and an understanding of both viewpoints is fundamental to the effective restoration of the partially dentate mouth. The following chapter is concerned mainly with the functional aspects of jaw relationships. For a detailed consideration of the anatomical and neuro-physiological aspects the reader is referred to standard textbooks.

Within the range of functional relationships between mandible and maxilla, it is important to separate the *non-contact* relationships, when the teeth are apart, from the *contact* relationships, when the teeth are together.

Non-contact relationships

The teeth are apart and the mandible moves entirely under the influence of the muscles of mastication and the articular surfaces of the temporomandibular joints *(posterior guidance)*.

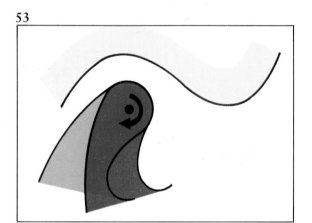

53 Movement within the temporomandibular joints can involve simple rotation of the condyle along the retruded arc of closure of the mandible. This arc, described by the mandible while the condyles are in their most posterior position, occurs over the last 20 mm of closure as measured from the lower mid-incisal point.

The axis of rotation through the condyles is known as the retruded hinge axis and it is often used for mounting casts on adjustable articulators as it is reproducible, being unaffected by loss of teeth or changes in the occlusal surfaces of the teeth.

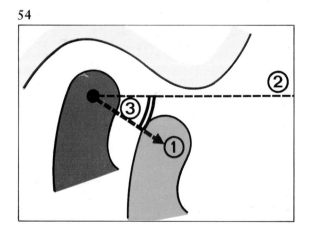

54 Condylar movement in protrusion involves translation of both condyles forward and downwards along the condylar path (1), establishing the posterior guidance. The condylar path is generally related to a horizontal plane of reference, the Frankfort plane (2), which passes through the superior margin of the external auditory canal and the inferior margin of the bony orbit. The angle (3) formed between this plane and the condylar path is the condylar or sagittal condylar angle.

55   In lateral excursion, one condyle moves downwards, forwards and medially and the angle which its path of movement makes with the sagittal plane is known as the Bennett angle (1). The other moves predominantly in the horizontal plane involving a combination of rotation and some degree of lateral translation (Bennett movement) of the mandible (2). The side towards which the mandible moves is described as the working side and the other as the non-working side.

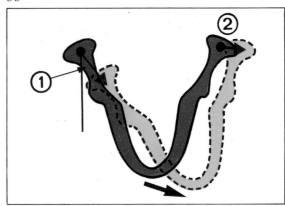

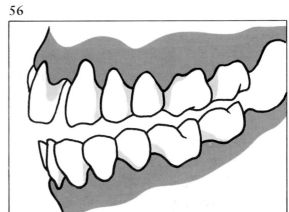

Rest position and freeway space

56   When the muscles of mastication are relaxed there is usually a space between upper and lower teeth. This is called the freeway space or interocclusal distance and when viewed in the sagittal plane is wedge-shaped, with a separation in the incisal region which is usually within the range 2–4 mm.

Contact relationships

Contact between the teeth of the opposing dental arches serves to control the amount of jaw separation and to have a moderating influence on the basic pattern of movement of the mandible (*anterior guidance*).

Intercuspal position (ICP)

57   This is the position of maximum intercuspation of the posterior teeth. In a stable occlusion it is characterised by simultaneous bilateral contact of several pairs of opposing posterior teeth with no discernible anteroposterior or lateral slide as the mandible closes under reflex muscular control. It is a position which patients should be able to find spontaneously and represents the closest relationship of mandible to maxilla when natural teeth are present.

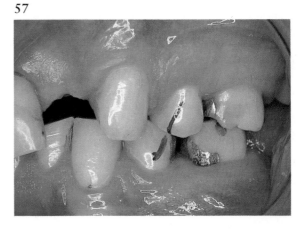

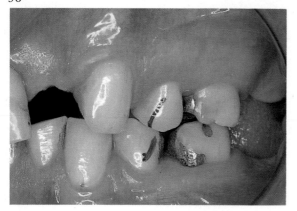

Retruded contact position

58 This is a contact relationship in which the mandible is located 1–1.5 mm distal to the intercuspal position. There are generally fewer tooth contacts present than in ICP and there is a slightly greater vertical separation of mandible from maxilla as the contact is on the slopes of the cusps. Ideally, movement from retruded contact to intercuspal position should be a forward slide with no lateral deviation.

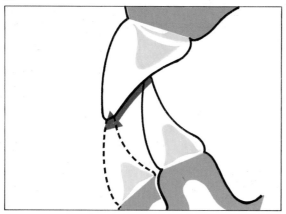

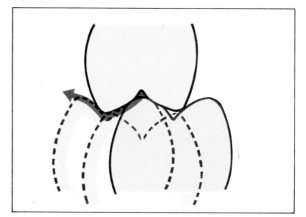

Protrusive relationship

59 Normally, protrusion of the mandible will lead initially to contact of the labial surfaces or incisal edges of the lower anterior teeth against the palatal aspect of the upper incisors and eventually to an edge-to-edge incisal contact.

Thus in this early stage of protrusion, the direction of mandibular movement is determined by the palatal slope of the upper incisors; this is known as incisal guidance. Commonly this movement is associated with separation of the posterior occlusal surfaces. Where the incisors commence in an edge-to-edge relationship or where the lower incisors are in advance of the uppers, protrusive movement will carry the lower incisors forward of the upper teeth, often with quite widespread contact of the posterior occlusal surfaces.

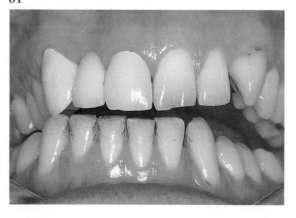

Lateral excursion

60 Cuspal inclines of posterior teeth influence the path of lateral excursion as shown here during movement of the mandible from ICP.

61 In lateral excursion, there will generally be contact of the opposing dentitions on the working side following one of two patterns.

Contact may be established almost immediately between the canines with separation of all the other teeth – a situation described as *canine guidance*.

62 Alternatively, contact may be maintained between a group of teeth, usually centred in the canine/premolar region, with gradual separation of the remaining teeth – a situation described as *group function*.

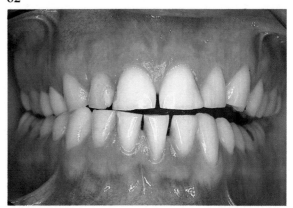

63 Generally there will be complete separation of the teeth on the non-working side and any isolated non-working side contact, such as between 15 and 46, should be regarded as a potential occlusal interference during such excursive movements. Occasionally there may be bilateral occlusal balance in the natural dentition similar to that described in complete denture construction.

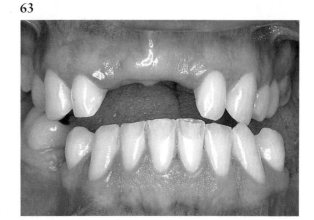

Contact movements are thus influenced both by posterior guidance from the temporo-mandibular joints and by anterior guidance from the teeth. It will be clear that it is the contact relationships which will be the determining factor in developing the occlusal scheme for most removable partial dentures.

64 The movement between the various contact relationships of the mandible is generally described as commencing in ICP with excursion out to a protruded or lateral position. This provides a convenient way of describing and analysing mandibular movement and such excursions are indeed characteristic of the parafunctional grinding and rubbing activity of bruxism. However, in masticatory function, the movement often takes place in the opposite direction. Closure through the bolus of food thus brings the mandible from the excursive position back to the intercuspal position.

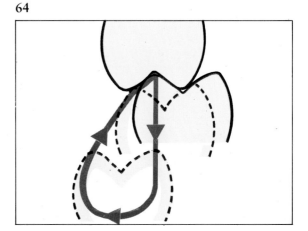

65 to 67 The total range of mandibular movement can be represented by a so-called *envelope of movement* traced by the mandibular mid-incisal point and described originally by Posselt. This envelope is shown in the sagittal plane (**65**), in the coronal plane (**66**) and in the horizontal plane (**67**).

65

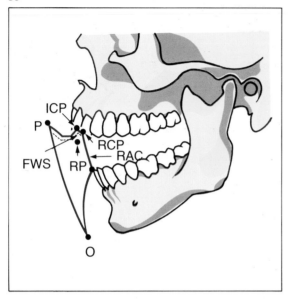

66

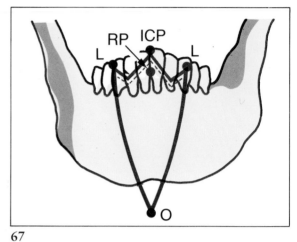

67

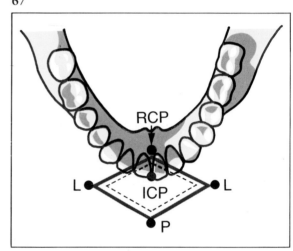

KEY

ICP	intercuspal position
RCP	retruded contact position
RAC	retruded arc of closure
RP	rest position
FWS	freeway space (judged to be the distance between the rest position and the intercuspal position).
P	maximum protrusion
O	maximum opening
L	maximum lateral excursion
- - - -	contact movements
———	non-contact movements

68 The extent to which these features of the various tooth contact relationships will influence partial denture design and construction will depend on the number and location of the missing teeth. With minimal tooth loss and a stable intercuspal relationship the occlusion of the partial denture should harmonise with the existing intercuspal relationship and with the various excursive guidances established by the remaining teeth.

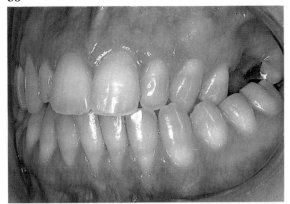

69 When loss of posterior teeth has eliminated the entire posterior occlusal table in one or both jaws there is no longer any record of the intercuspal position. In these circumstances the horizontal jaw relationship should be recorded in the retruded position. The occlusal vertical relationship is derived from the resting vertical dimension after making an allowance for an appropriate freeway space. The prosthetic occlusion is thus established in the retruded jaw relationship and the intercuspal position is then identical with the retruded contact position. However, it will usually be necessary to equilibrate the occlusion to allow some forward slide to take place.

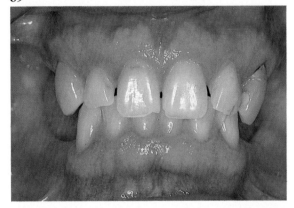

70 Problems can also arise when tooth loss and occlusal wear are superimposed on an underlying malocclusion. Here, the initial contact takes place in the anterior region and the occlusal surfaces of the posterior teeth are separated by at least 2 mm.

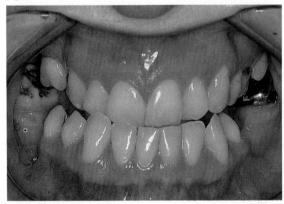

71 The mandible has now been guided forward into a position of accommodation in which there is contact of the posterior teeth and a reverse incisal overbite of about 2 mm.

If this pattern of occlusal contact is left uncorrected there is a danger that individual teeth will become functionally overloaded with risk of excessive tooth wear or periodontal breakdown. It is also possible that the patient may develop mandibular dysfunction, as indeed happened in this instance.

In these circumstances it will be necessary to record the retruded jaw relationship on the retruded arc of closure, to undertake equilibration of the teeth and to provide a partial lower denture with occlusal overlays to establish stable contact in this position.

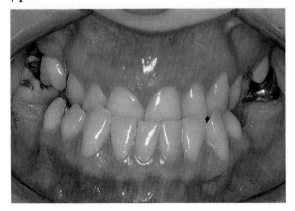

4 History and examination

The aim of recording the history and under-taking the clinical examination is to collect those facts which will help in establishing a diagnosis of any presenting problems and to formulate a treatment plan.

In assessing the possible requirement for partial dentures it is always important to bear in mind the patient's reason for seeking dental treatment and the level of motivation towards the maintenance of oral hygiene. It is also helpful to note whether or not the patient is actively seeking the provision of a partial denture or dentures.

72

```
                REASON FOR ATTENDANCE
    PDH ─────────────┐            PMH
                     ↓           ╱
                  HISTORY ◄──────
    ATTITUDE ────────╱
                     │
                     ↓
                EXAMINATION
                     │
                     ↓
                 DIAGNOSIS
                     │
                     ↓
              TREATMENT PLAN
```

72 The previous dental and medical histories may influence the patient's attitude to dental treat-ment. Because they are also likely to have had some effect on the current status of the dentition and on the ability and willingness of the patient to co-operate in oral hygiene and maintenance procedures, they must be taken into account when establishing a treatment plan. The accompanying flow chart illustrates the interaction of these various factors which will now be considered in greater detail.

Previous dental history

It is important to record details of previous dental treatment, to pay particular attention to any favourable or unfavourable comments on partial dentures which may have been provided in the past, and to assess the com-ments in relation to the suitability of any partial denture which is being worn at the time of the examination. These may prove to be particularly helpful in establishing the design of a replacement prosthesis.

Previous medical history

A detailed and accurate medical history is an essential requirement in the planning of any form of dental treatment. There are very few absolute contra-indications to the provision of partial dentures but the patient's general health should be carefully assessed, particularly in so far as it may affect the ability of the patient to maintain an adequate standard of oral and denture hygiene and to cope with the wearing of the prosthesis. It is important also to note details of drugs which the patient may be taking, as many therapeutic agents can have side effects in the oral cavity. For example, certain anti-depressants reduce salivary flow, creating problems in oral and denture hygiene. It may also be necessary to institute drug treatment during dental procedures, as, for example, the administration of antibiotics as a prophylactic measure against subacute bacterial endocarditis. Problems can arise because of the damage that a partial denture may cause in the mouth in the presence of lowered tissue resistance brought about by anaemia, diabetes or immuno-suppression. In some circumstances, it may be wiser to defer dental treatment until there has been an improvement in health or to provide a simple transitional denture as an interim measure.

Examination

Extra-oral

73a and **73b** Examination should begin with an extra-oral assessment of facial form and symmetry, a study of jaw opening and closing movements, together with palpation of the temporomandibular joints and muscles of mastication. The information derived from these observations is helpful in the assessment of the health of the masticatory system. The deviation of this patient's mandible to the left on closing indicates possible disharmony which should be investigated.

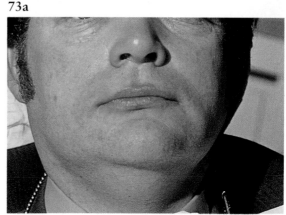

73a

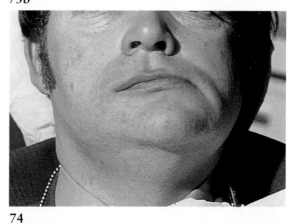

73b

Intra-oral

74 Preliminary visual inspection of the mouth will indicate the basic standard of oral hygiene, the level of caries susceptibility and the quality of the existing restorations. Special attention should be directed to any areas of specific complaint and it may be necessary to institute emergency treatment for the relief of pain. In this instance there is a need to improve the standard of oral hygiene and to replace a number of the existing restorations.

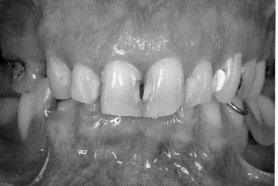

74

75 Detailed examination should commence with the soft tissues. The mucosa of the lips, cheeks, tongue, palate and floor of the mouth should be examined and tongue movements observed in order to exclude pathology. Here, the mucosa appears to be normal.

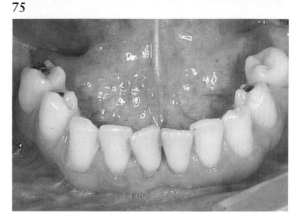

75

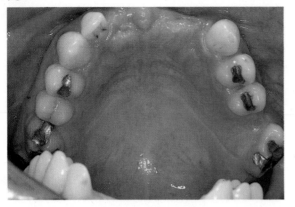

76 The individual dental arches should be carefully inspected, the location of edentulous spaces noted and the distribution and alignment of the remaining teeth carefully assessed in relation to these spaces. Here there has been virtually no movement of the teeth adjacent to the anterior edentulous area; adequate space is available for the three replacement teeth. The same cannot be said of the molar space, which has been markedly reduced by rotation of 27.

77

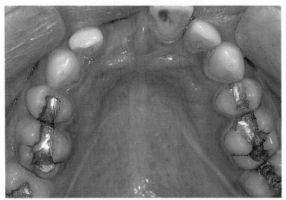

77 The presence of gingival or mucosal inflammation in an area covered by a previous denture should be noted so that appropriate treatment may be initiated.

78

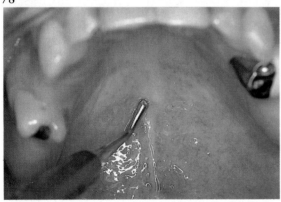

78 The form of the residual ridges and the compressibility of the investing soft tissues in the edentulous areas should be assessed visually and by palpation. Included in this examination is the hard palate since incompressible areas may have to be avoided by denture margins.

79

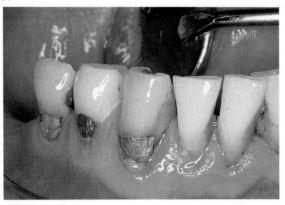

79 The integrity of existing restorations should be carefully checked and carious cavities charted.

80 The health of the periodontal tissues should be determined.

The standard of plaque control should be assessed and disclosing agents may be used to demonstrate the presence of plaque to the patient; plaque scores may be recorded.

Pocket depth should be measured and charted. Any mobility of the remaining teeth should be noted, especially if they are potential abutment teeth.

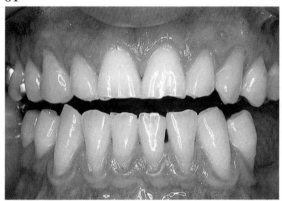

The dental arches should then be examined in occlusion and a very critical assessment made of the stability of the occlusion. Closure into the intercuspal position should be an automatic reflex procedure. Ideally, simultaneous bilateral contact should take place. Any contact which disturbs this pattern should be noted, particularly if it gives rise to displacement of the mandible into a position of accommodation.

81 In this mouth the initial contact on closure takes place between the canine teeth on the right side.

81

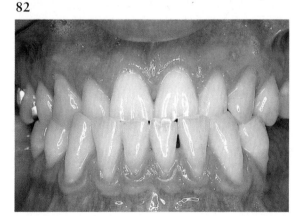

82

82 The mandible has now been guided forward into a postural position in which there is substantial contact between the opposing dentitions in the anterior and posterior regions.

Before a treatment plan is established, it must be decided whether the existing occlusal relationship should be accepted or whether it should be modified, either by equilibration to eliminate the initial canine contact or by reconstructing the deficient posterior occlusion at the occlusal vertical dimension established by the initial contact.

83

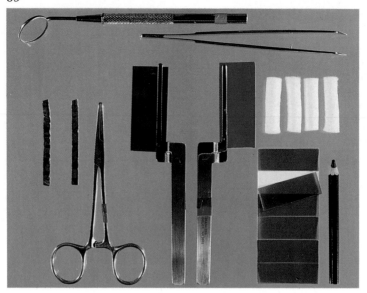

83 Occlusal indicator wax, articulating paper or tape, and thin metal foil (shimstock) as shown here may be helpful in clinical assessment of the occlusion. It is also helpful to mount study casts on an articulator.

84

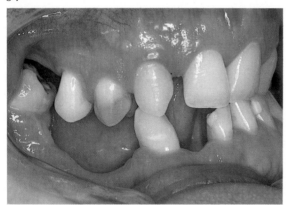

84 Any drifting or tilting of teeth which may have been noted when the individual dental arches were examined should be reassessed in relation to the opposing arch. The abnormal position may contribute to occlusal faults or to problems when designing a denture in the other jaw. Overerupted teeth, such as 14, 15 and 47, should also be noted as remedial treatment in the form of occlusal equilibration or even reduction in height and restoration by means of crowns may be required.

85

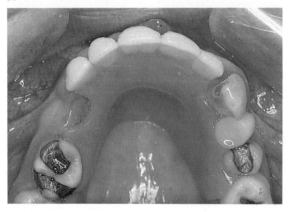

85 Existing partial dentures should be examined. The design and quality of construction should be noted and any associated problems in relation to gingival and mucosal inflammation or to decalcification of contacting tooth surfaces carefully evaluated. It is important to assess whether or not the denture still fits accurately against the teeth and the underlying mucosa. The appearance of the denture should also be noted.

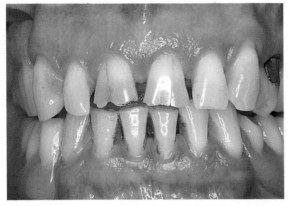

86 The degree to which the denture restores occlusal contact should be assessed. Here, alveolar resorption and occlusal wear of the artificial teeth have resulted in lack of posterior tooth contact, causing increased loading on the anterior teeth.

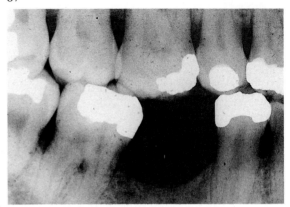

87 Radiographs should be obtained to check for new or recurrent carious lesions which may not have been revealed by clinical inspection, to reveal the extent of any bone loss which may be present and also to identify any pathological changes within the jaws.

The quality of the existing restorations and the degree of bone loss in the interproximal areas can be assessed from this bite-wing radiograph.

Diagnosis

If the reason for the patient's initial attendance was centred on a complaint, then the penultimate stage of the history and examination phase is to establish a diagnosis from which will stem the treatment plan. Complaints will come in many forms and may be related to such things as pain in the teeth, facial pain, difficulty in eating, a deteriorating appearance or an existing partial denture which is unsatisfactory. Whatever the complaint, it is important that the findings from the history, the examination and any special tests provide sufficient evidence for the cause to be established.

Treatment plan

Any necessary emergency treatment should be undertaken. Impressions should be recorded and study casts obtained and if necessary mounted on an articulator. An initial treatment plan should then be drawn up and discussed with the patient as it may often be necessary for this treatment to be phased over a number of interim stages prior to establishing a definitive treatment plan.

The permutation of treatment plans for individual patients is enormous. Alternatives could range from fixed restorations to precision attachments or even to extraction of the remaining teeth and the provision of complete dentures. It is not the purpose of this Atlas to consider these alternatives in any detail but rather to look at the management of those patients for whom a removable partial denture is to be provided.

Part 3 explains in greater detail the treatment procedures involved in the preparation of the mouth for partial dentures.

The sequence of treatment will usually be dictated by the severity of carious attack and periodontal involvement, but it is essential to establish a provisional denture design at this early stage so that the treatment which follows may be undertaken in the most logical order and be planned with the denture design already in mind. For instance, the contours of crowns should be planned to provide, where required, guiding surfaces, rest seat preparations and suitable undercuts for clasps.

Decisions on what is required and the correct sequence for the individual patient can only be made at the chairside.

5 Preliminary impressions

Preliminary impressions of a patient's mouth are obtained in stock, 'off-the-peg', impression trays. The resulting study casts are needed for planning treatment, including the designing of partial dentures, and for the construction of individual trays which will be used to obtain the more accurate working impressions required for the construction of the partial dentures.

88

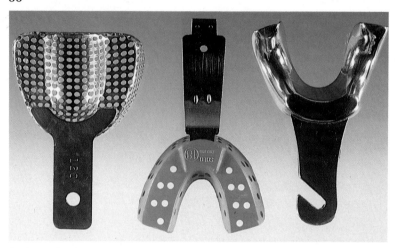

88 Stock trays are available in a variety of sizes and shapes. They may be perforated or un-perforated, metal or plastic, of simple box design or shaped to fit bilateral free-end saddles.

89

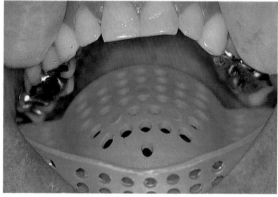

89 A size of tray is selected so that the teeth sit centrally within the trough of the tray. If possible there should be a space of about 4 mm between the flange of the tray and the buccal and labial surfaces of the teeth.

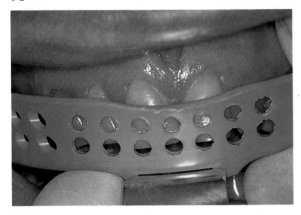

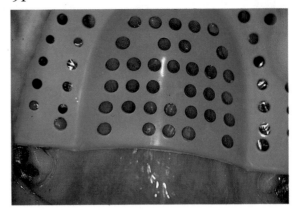

90 and **91** Because the range of stock trays is limited it will commonly be found that an ideal size and shape of stock tray is not available. In this example, the upper stock tray does not cover the labial surfaces of the teeth sufficiently, neither does it include the most posterior teeth.

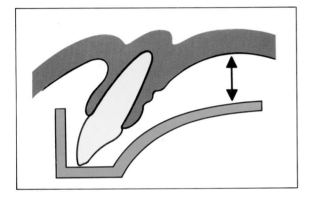

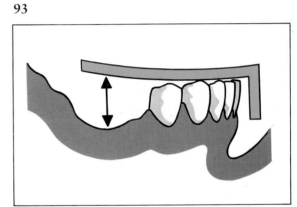

92 and **93** There may also be regions where the tray is poorly adapted to the underlying structures such as the palate or a saddle area.

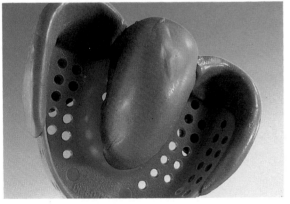

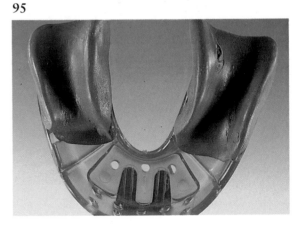

94 and **95** In each case the dead space should be filled by placing impression compound in the appropriate area. The compound will then be moulded in the mouth.

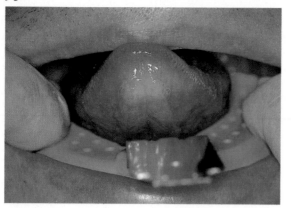

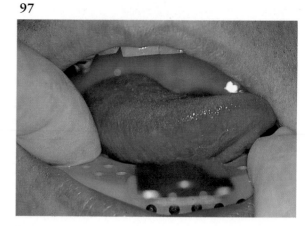

96 and 97 Lingual border moulding of the compound is achieved by the patient first pushing the tongue to contact the upper lip – and then thrusting the tongue into each corner of the mouth in turn.

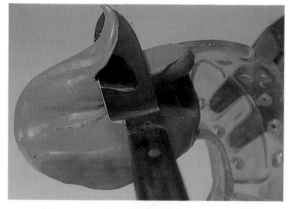

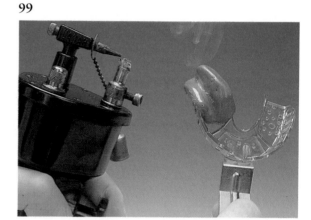

98 and 99 Any areas of the impression compound which are overextended should be corrected by trimming away the excess material, resoftening in a flame and tempering in warm water before repeating the border moulding.

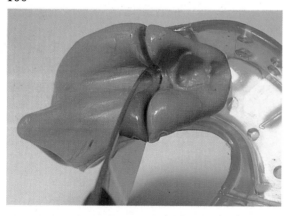

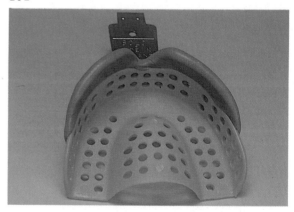

100 Compound that has contacted the teeth should be cut away as it may prevent accurate reinsertion of the impression tray and will eliminate space around the teeth necessary for a sufficient thickness of the alginate used to complete the preliminary impression.

101 Underextension in the labial region can be corrected by the addition of impression compound to the deficient areas of the tray to form a slightly overextended flange.

102 The tray is then seated in the mouth while the compound is still soft and border moulding is carried out. Buccal and labial moulding of both upper and lower impressions is achieved by supporting the tray with one hand while manipulating the cheeks and lips with the other.

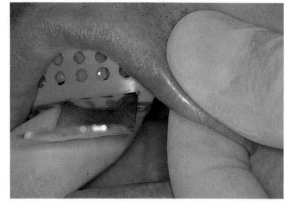

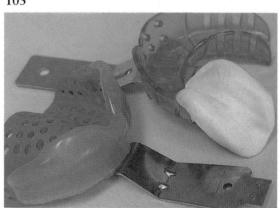

103

103 When a water bath is not available for softening the impression compound, alternative materials, such as silicone putty or pink modelling wax, may be used to modify the tray. However, silicone putty is more expensive than impression compound whilst wax is more easily deformed at mouth temperature.

Once modification of the stock tray has been completed any additions of compound are thoroughly chilled and the tray is dried. A thin layer of adhesive is applied and allowed to dry before the tray is loaded with alginate. The tray is then seated in the mouth and the impression material border-moulded.

104

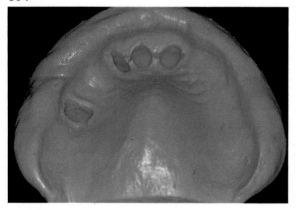

105

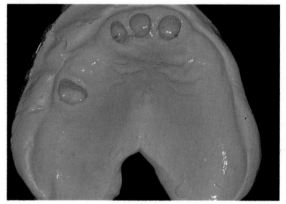

104 and **105** The completed impression is assessed by considering three aspects:

    1 those sulcus areas which will be related to the denture borders,

    2 the saddle areas,

    3 the teeth.

The impression on the left is satisfactory, the one on the right shows a number of faults: the tray has been positioned too far to the patient's left, the borders of the alginate are unsupported and the impression is underextended in the post-dam region.

If on inspection the impression is found to be satisfactory, it is rinsed thoroughly to remove all traces of saliva and may be dipped in a disinfectant. The impression should be rinsed again and shaken to remove any excess moisture.

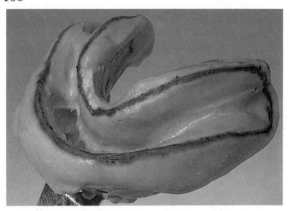

106 An indelible pencil line may be drawn on the impression to indicate to the technician the required extension of the individual tray.

The completed impression must be prevented from drying out by covering it with a damp gauze and placing it in a plastic bag.

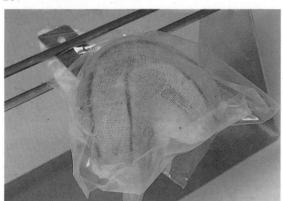

107 While the impression is waiting to be cast the tray should be supported so that its own weight is not applied to the borders of the impression. If this is not done, permanent deformation of the impression will occur.

The impression must be cast as soon as possible to avoid inaccuracies developing as a result of the dimensional instability of alginate.

The instructions to the laboratory should include details of the type of individual tray required for the working impressions (Chapter 22).

6 Articulators

An articulator is a hinge-like device which can be used to position the upper and lower casts in a chosen relationship to each other. There are many different designs of articulator, several of which reproduce some of the movements of which the mandible is capable.

Types of articulator

Hinge articulator

108 This simple articulator holds the casts in a prescribed relationship, usually the intercuspal position, and allows separation and approximation of the casts. The hinge is in no way related to the hinge axis of the mandible and there is no attempt to reproduce mandibular movement. Thus with this type of articulator it is possible to produce even occlusal contact only in the recorded static jaw relationship. The limitations of this device have long been recognised.

If this instrument is used at all it must be in circumstances where the occlusion is to be restored to an existing stable intercuspal relationship and where the excursive guidances of the remaining natural teeth will ensure separation of those teeth replaced by the partial denture.

It will also be necessary to identify and eliminate occlusal discrepancies when the restoration is inserted in the mouth.

Average movement articulator

109 Articulators of this type have their origins in the work of Monson, Bonwill and Gysi, who recorded measurements from anatomical specimens and clinical subjects in order to develop articulators whose dimensions reflected those anatomical features which influence mandibular movement. The dimensions of these articulators reflect the average measurement recorded by Bonwill of 10 cm between the central points of the mandibular condyles and between these points and the midpoint of the incisal edges of the lower anterior teeth. These dimensions form an equilateral triangle, known as Bonwill's triangle.

110 These articulators also incorporate a condylar path representing the average sagittal condylar guidance angle of approximately 30°.

The maxillary cast is mounted in its correct position relative to the condylar axis by means of a locating device such as an incisal pin, or in some instances by the use of a facebow (**113**). This group of arbitrary movement articulators is widely used in dental practice but clearly has limitations in its capacity to replicate mandibular movement.

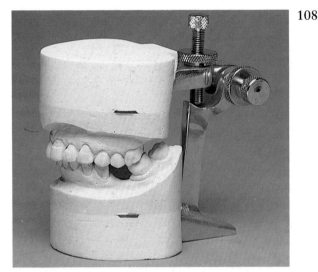

108

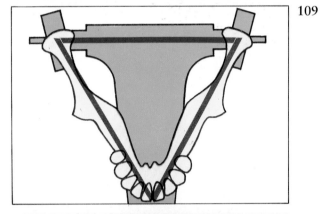

109

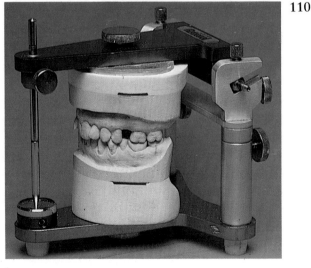

110

Semi-adjustable articulators

In order to reproduce the mandibular movements of individual patients with any degree of accuracy, articulators need to be adjustable to conform to those anatomical features, such as incisal guidance and condylar guidance, which influence those movements and to take account of the bodily shift of the mandible (Bennett movement) during lateral excursion.

Two basic types of adjustable articulators are available, both of which produce a reasonable simulation of anatomical relationships and movements, which allow satisfactory occlusal function to be restored in a wide variety of clinical situations.

111

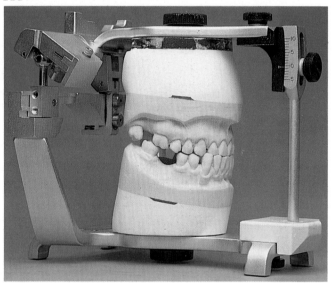

Arcon type
(mandibulAR CONdyle)

111 Articulators of the arcon type, such as the Whipmix and Denar series, have a condylar element on the lower member which is able to slide against an adjustable plane on the maxillary component of the articulator. A Denar instrument is illustrated here.

112

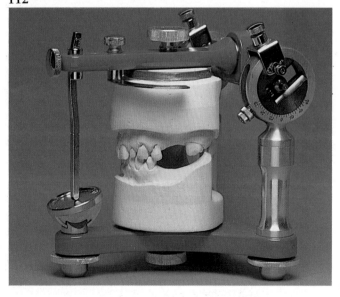

Non-Arcon type

112 In this group of articulators, like the Dentatus Type ARL illustrated here, the condylar sphere is part of the upper member of the articulator and is contained within an adjustable track in the condylar pillar of the lower element.

Records required for semi-adjustable articulators

Facebow transfer

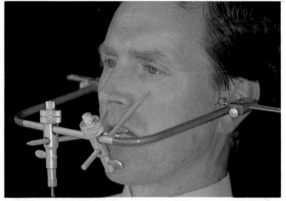

113a and 113b A prerequisite of all adjustable articulators is that the cast of the maxillary dentition should be located accurately in relation to the mandibular condyles and to a horizontal plane of reference, usually the Frankfort plane. A facebow is used to record this information clinically (**a**) and to transfer it to the articulator (**b**).

Occlusal records

113b

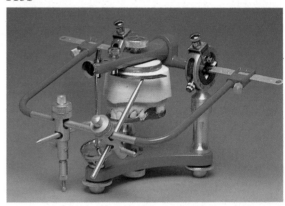

If the intercuspal relationship is comfortable and well defined it should be accepted, particularly if excursive guidances are established by the natural dentition. If all the remaining posterior teeth occlude very precisely it may be possible to locate the casts in the intercuspal position. The casts must then be securely located together before being mounted on the articulator. Alternatively the relationship may be recorded using a wax template shaped as in **114**.

114

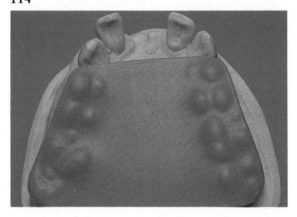

114 If there is a deviation on closing from the first contact position to intercuspal position, it is essential to analyse the occlusion and locate the interference. In these circumstances it is advisable to obtain a record of the retruded jaw relationship just prior to tooth contact. The recording template is made from two thicknesses of toughened wax. It is usually advisable to trim the template to avoid incisal contact. A horseshoe shape is not sufficiently rigid. The wax is softened, placed in the mouth and the mandible guided into closure along the retruded hinge axis. Tooth-to-tooth contact through this wax must be avoided as this may cause deviation of the mandible.

115

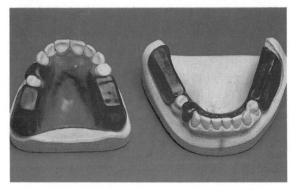

115 If there are insufficient teeth remaining for a record of this type to be used successfully, it will be necessary to construct wax occlusal rims. These are adjusted in the mouth to record the prescribed jaw relationship, as described in Chapter 23.

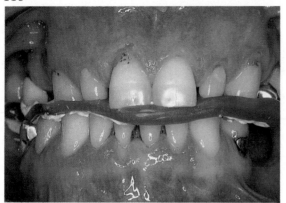

116 When an adjustable articulator is to be used it is necessary to prepare wax indices to record the jaw relationship in protrusive or in right and left lateral excursions. These indices are used to set the condylar guidance angles on the articulator.

Here is an example of a record of a right lateral excursion. In this particular instance the accuracy of the tooth indentations has been increased by using registration paste on the wax wafer.

117

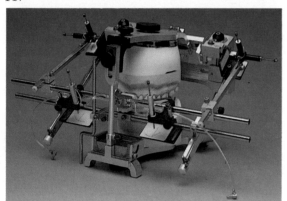

Fully adjustable articulators

117 These are sophisticated articulators with a more comprehensive system of adjustment which gives them the potential for increased accuracy in the reproduction of mandibular movement. Various methods have been devised for programming these instruments, for example, by obtaining tracings of mandibular movement in three planes using an instrument called a pantograph and then transferring these records to the articulator.

Their use demands a high degree of skill on the part of the clinical and technical personnel and the clinical procedures are time-consuming.

Part 2
Partial denture design

A partial denture is the sum of a number of individual components. In this part of the Atlas we discuss the functions and construction of the various components before describing a system of design.

7 Classification of the partially edentulous arch

A classification to describe and simplify the almost infinite variety of permutations of teeth and edentulous areas is desirable. It facilitates the recording of case histories and aids discussion between clinicians and communication with technicians. It may also allow the clinician to anticipate the basic type of partial denture design that is appropriate for a particular patient.

Classifications in current use are of two types – those which classify the partial denture and those which classify the partially edentulous arch.

118a to **118c** An example of a classification which describes partial dentures is based on the nature of the support utilised by a partial denture. Support can be gained from:

(**a**) teeth,

(**b**) mucosa,

(**c**) teeth and mucosa.

This concept is discussed in more detail in Chapter 10. The virtue of this classification is that it focuses attention on the problem of support, which is a very important factor in partial denture design. However, it does not convey any information about the number and distribution of the edentulous spaces and it is largely for this reason that a greater popularity is enjoyed by the more descriptive classification which follows.

118a

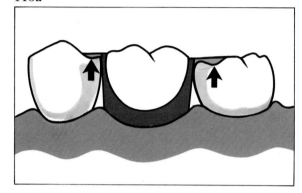

118b

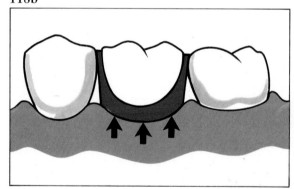

118c

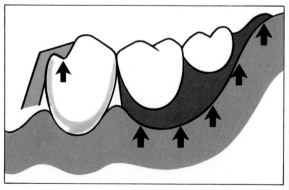

Of the classifications which describe the partially edentulous arch the most widely used is that introduced by Kennedy in 1928.

This is an anatomical classification which describes the number and distribution of edentulous areas present.

119

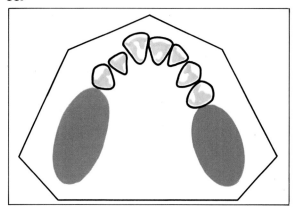

119   Class I: bilateral edentulous areas located posterior to the remaining natural teeth. Denture saddles which restore such edentulous areas are described as 'free-end saddles'.

120

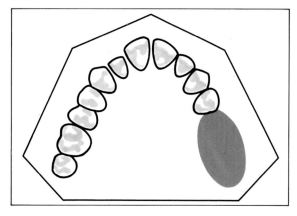

120   Class II: a unilateral edentulous area located posterior to the remaining natural teeth.

121

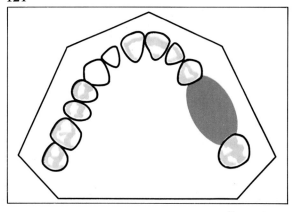

121   Class III: a unilateral edentulous area with natural teeth remaining both anterior and posterior to it. Denture saddles which restore this type of edentulous area are said to be 'bounded saddles'.

123   In Classes I–III any additional edentulous area is referred to as a Modification. This example would be described as Class III Modification 2 (there being two additional edentulous areas).

122

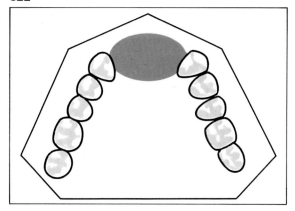

122   Class IV: a single edentulous area located anterior to the remaining natural teeth.

123

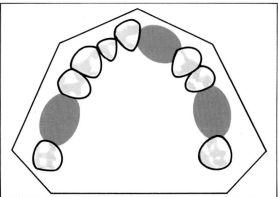

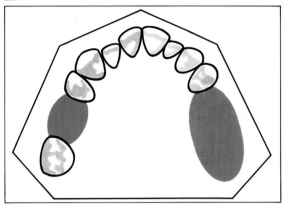

124 The classification is always determined by the most posterior edentulous area. For example, the classification of the arch illustrated is determined by the presence of the free-end saddle area, not by the bounded saddle area. This example is therefore a Kennedy Class II Modification 1.

Because of this principle there can be no modifications to the Kennedy Class IV arch.

Classification of an arch helps to direct the clinician's thoughts to the problems which are characteristic of the class and thus to the broad principles of design which are likely to be appropriate. The main problems are outlined below. The solutions are described more fully in the relevant sections of the Atlas.

125

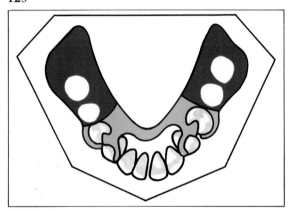

126

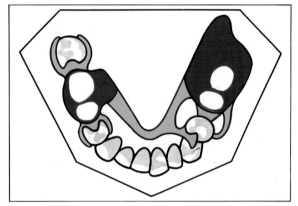

125 Kennedy Class I. The absence of abutment teeth distally creates problems both of support and retention.

The problem of support arises from the fact that the abutment tooth offers firmer support than the mucosa of the edentulous area. Great care must be taken in the design and construction of the denture to minimise the undesirable effects of this support differential.

The other major problem is that there are no teeth posteriorly to retain the saddle against movement in an occlusal direction. Specific measures must be employed to prevent this movement. These will include utilising the principle of indirect retention (Chapter 13), here illustrated by placing incisal rests on 33 and 43, and correct shaping of the buccal and lingual polished surfaces of the saddles to assist neuromuscular control.

126 Kennedy Class II. Like the Class I arch this requires a denture which is both tooth- and mucosa-supported but in this instance there is often a modification present which can be tooth-supported. Once again there is the opportunity for the free-end saddle to move but the situation is not so critical because there are teeth on the other side of the arch with the potential to provide more effective retention.

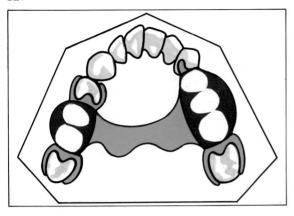

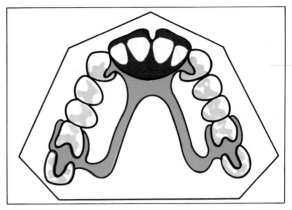

127 Kennedy Class III. In this situation there is the opportunity for the denture to be entirely supported and retained by teeth. Therefore the difficulties in producing a stable denture are likely to be less than for Classes I and II. However, it will be appreciated that complications will arise when one or more of the abutment teeth cannot be clasped because of an unsuitable contour or because a clasp would detract from the appearance, as would be the case for 23 in the illustration. Under such circumstances indirect retention will be required.

If the denture does not replace a large number of teeth and is fully tooth-supported the connector can be reduced in size as it will not have a supportive function.

128 Kennedy Class IV. Appearance is of paramount importance in this class. As a consequence it is rarely possible to clasp the abutment teeth. Therefore alternative means of retaining the saddle need to be sought, including the use of a labial flange. In addition the retentive clasps must be located with great care so that the benefits of indirect retention can be realised, in this instance by placing extended rests on 17 and 27.

8 Surveying

129 The surveyor was first introduced to the dental profession in 1918. This instrument, which is essentially a parallelometer, is one of the cornerstones of effective partial denture design and construction. The surveyor allows a vertical arm to be brought into contact with the teeth and ridges of the dental cast, thus identifying parallel surfaces and points of maximum contour.

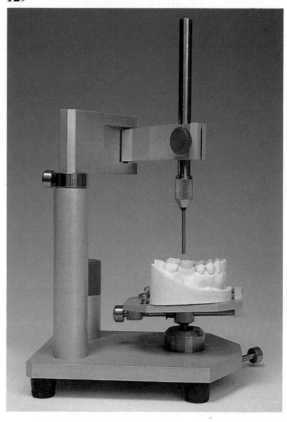

129

It is the clinician's responsibility to survey the study cast and then use the information obtained to design the partial denture. It is this design, produced in the light of clinical knowledge and experience, which guides decisions on pre-prosthetic treatment and which is ultimately sent as a prescription to the dental technician, who constructs the denture accordingly.

There are several different attachments which may be used with the surveyor:

Analysing rod

130 This metal rod is placed against the teeth and ridges during the initial analysis of the cast to identify undercut areas and to determine the parallelism of surfaces without marking the cast.

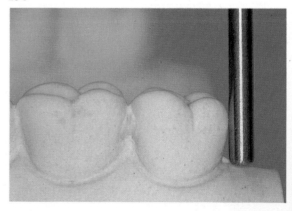

130

Graphite marker

131 The graphite marker is moved around the tooth and along the alveolar ridge to identify and mark the position of maximum convexity (SURVEY LINE) separating non-undercut from undercut areas.

When surveying a tooth, the tip of the marker should be level with the gingival margin allowing the *side* of the marker to produce the survey line as shown in the illustration.

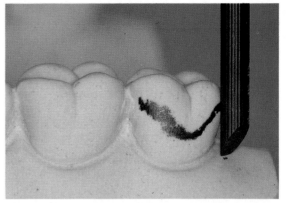

132 A false survey line will be produced if the tip of the marker is incorrectly positioned. In this example there is not, in fact, an undercut area on the tooth although an incorrect surveying technique has indicated one. If this false line is used in designing a partial denture, errors will arise in the positioning of components, especially clasps.

132

Undercut gauge

133 Gauges are provided to measure the extent of horizontal undercut and are available in the following sizes: 0.25 mm, 0.50 mm and 0.75 mm. By adjusting the vertical position of the gauge until the shank and head contact the cast simultaneously, the point at which a specific extent of horizontal undercut occurs can be identified and marked. This procedure allows correct positioning of retentive clasp arms on the tooth surface as described in Chapter 11.

Other, more sophisticated, types of undercut gauge are available such as dial gauges and electronic gauges. These attachments fulfil the same function as the simpler type of gauge.

133

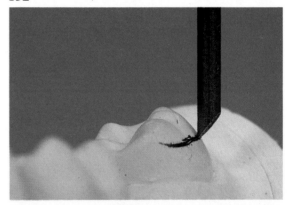

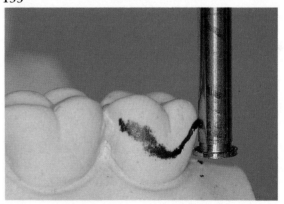

Trimming knife

134 This instrument is used to eliminate unwanted undercuts on the master cast. Wax is added to these unwanted undercut areas and then the excess is removed with the trimmer so that the modified surfaces are parallel to the chosen path of insertion. A duplicate cast is then made on which the denture is manufactured. Such a procedure eliminates the problem shown in **135**.

When elimination of undercuts is required on a cast which is not to be duplicated a material such as zinc phosphate cement, which can resist the boiling out procedure, is employed. The surveyor is used to shape the cement before it is fully set.

134

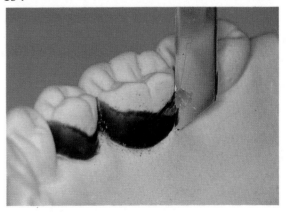

135a

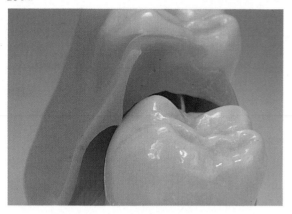

135b

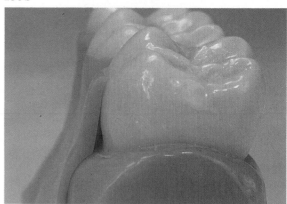

135a This partial denture cannot be inserted in the mouth because failure to eliminate unwanted undercut on the cast has resulted in acrylic resin being processed into the area.

135b This denture has been processed on a correctly prepared cast and, as a result, there is no interference with insertion.

136

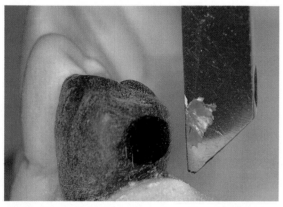

136 The trimming knife can also be used to prepare guide surfaces on wax patterns of crowns for abutment teeth (**137**).

Before discussing the functions of a surveyor in more detail it is necessary to explain the following terms:

Guide surfaces (or guide planes)

137

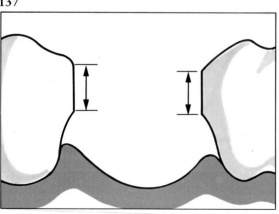

137 Two or more parallel axial surfaces on abutment teeth which can be used to limit the path of insertion (see page 59) and improve the stability of a removable prosthesis. Guide surfaces may occur naturally on teeth but will more commonly need to be prepared.

Path of insertion

The path followed by the denture from its first contact with the teeth until it is fully seated. This path coincides with the path of withdrawal and may or may not coincide with the path of displacement (see **143**). There may be a single path or multiple paths of insertion:

138

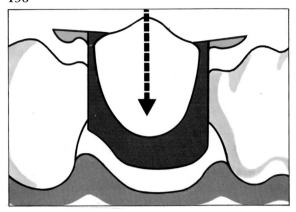

139

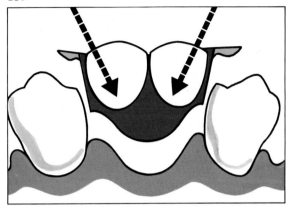

138 A *single* path of insertion may be created if sufficient guide surfaces are contacted by the denture; it is most likely to exist when bounded saddle areas are present.

139 *Multiple* paths of insertion will exist where guide surfaces are not utilised, for example where the abutment teeth are divergent.

140

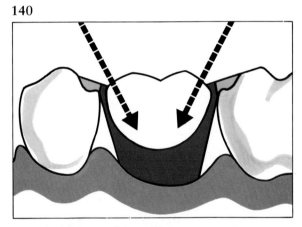

141

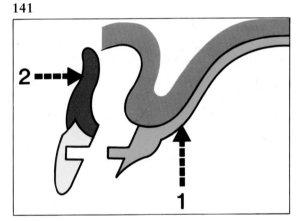

140 Multiple paths will also exist where point contact between the saddle of the denture and the abutment teeth is employed in the 'open' design of saddle. The philosophy for this approach is discussed in Chapter 9.

141 Two distinct paths of insertion will be employed for a sectional, or two-part denture illustrated here by a diagram in the sagittal plane of a Kennedy class IV denture. The abutment teeth on either side of the saddle are not shown.

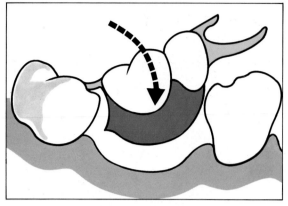

142 Occasionally a rotational path of insertion can be used.

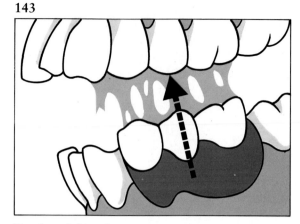

Path of displacement

143 This is the direction in which the denture tends to be displaced in function. The path is variable but is assumed for the purpose of design to be at right angles to the occlusal plane.

Surveying procedure

This may be divided into the following distinct phases:

1 preliminary visual assessment of the study cast,
2 initial survey,
3 analysis,
4 final survey.

Preliminary visual assessment of the study cast

This stage has been described as 'eyeballing' the cast and is a useful preliminary to the surveying procedure proper. The cast is held in the hand and inspected from above. The general form and arrangement of the teeth and ridge can be observed, any obvious problems noted and an idea obtained as to whether or not a tilted survey should be employed.

144

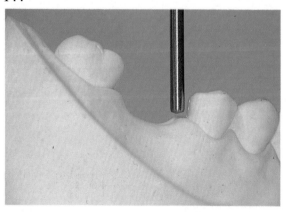

145

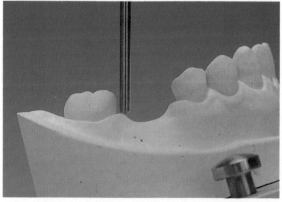

144 shows an anterior tilt ('heels up') and **145** a posterior tilt ('heels down'). Clinical experience indicates that these are the positions of the cast which most commonly give the greatest benefit. However, a lateral tilt of the cast to right or left may also be indicated on occasion.

Initial survey

146 The cast is positioned with the occlusal plane horizontal and then the teeth and ridges are surveyed to identify undercut areas which might be utilised to provide retention in relation to the most likely path of displacement.

The position of the survey lines and the variations in the horizontal extent of undercut associated with them should be noted. The amount of undercut can be judged approximately from the size of the 'triangle of light' between the marker and the cervical part of the tooth or measured more precisely by using an undercut gauge. An assessment can then be made as to whether the horizontal extent of undercut is sufficient for retention purposes.

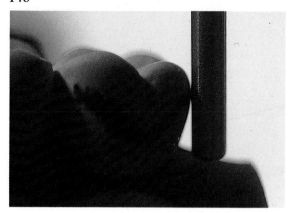

Analysis

A partial denture can be designed on a cast which has been surveyed with the occlusal plane horizontal (i.e. so that the path of insertion = the path of displacement). However, there are occasions when tilting of the cast is indicated so that the paths of insertion and displacement differ.

Before deciding if the cast should be tilted for the final survey the graphite marker in the surveyor is changed for an analysing rod so that various positions of the cast can be examined without marking the teeth.

The analysis of the cast continues with the occlusal plane horizontal and the following aspects, one or more of which might necessitate a final survey with the cast tilted, are considered:

1 appearance,
2 interference,
3 retention.

147

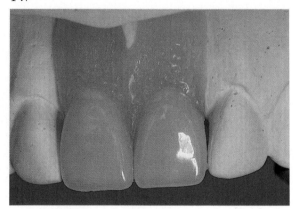

Appearance

147 When a maxillary cast, containing an anterior edentulous area, is surveyed with the occlusal plane horizontal it will often be found that there are undercuts on the mesial aspects of the abutment teeth.

If the partial denture is constructed with this vertical path of insertion there will be an unsightly gap between the denture saddle and the abutment teeth gingival to the contact point.

148

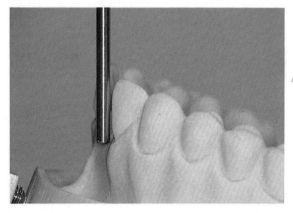

148 This unsightly gap can be avoided by giving the cast a posterior tilt so that the analysing rod is parallel with the mesiolabial surface of the abutment tooth.

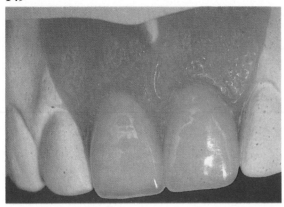

149 With this path of insertion the saddle can be made to contact the abutment tooth over the whole of the mesiolabial surface and a much better appearance results.

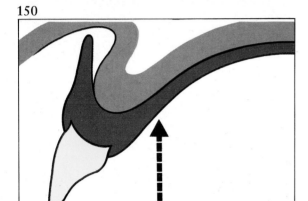

Interference

150 While examining the cast with the occlusal plane horizontal, it sometimes becomes apparent that an undercut tooth or ridge would obstruct the insertion and correct placement of a rigid part of the denture. By tilting the cast, a path of insertion may be found which avoids this interference. For example, if a bony undercut is present labially, insertion of a flanged denture along a path at right angles to the occlusal plane will only be possible if the flange stands away from the mucosa or is finished short of the undercut area. This can result in poor retention as well as a poor appearance.

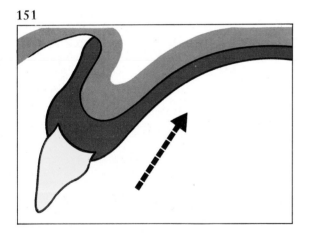

151 If the cast is given a posterior tilt so that the rod, and thus the path of insertion, is parallel to the labial surface of the ridge it is possible to insert a flange which fits the ridge accurately.

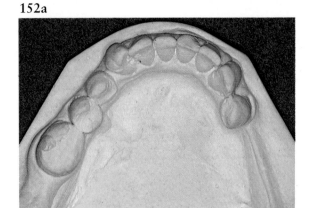

152a Lingually tilted premolars can make it impossible to place a sublingual, or lingual, bar connector sufficiently close to the lingual mucosa. Such a problem would occur lingually to 44.

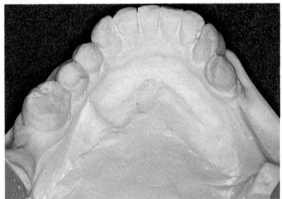

152b Giving the cast an anterior tilt reveals a path of insertion which avoids this interference.

If interference from a tooth is present and cannot be avoided by selecting an appropriate path of insertion, consideration should be given to the possibility of eliminating the interference by tooth preparation, for example by crowning to reduce the lingual overhang.

Retention

153 To obtain retention, undercuts *must* be present on teeth relative to the horizontal survey. It is a misconception to believe that changing the tilt of the cast will produce retentive undercuts if none exist when the cast is horizontal.

153

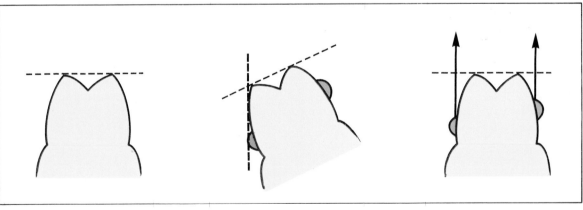

No undercuts on the tooth when the occlusal plane is horizontal.

An apparent undercut created by tilting the cast laterally. Clasp arms placed in this false undercut. . .

. . . do not provide any resistance to movement along the path of displacement.

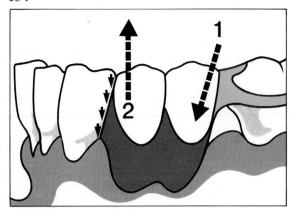

154 The principle of tilting the cast to enhance retention is that by so altering the path of insertion (1) a rigid part of the denture can enter an area of the tooth surface or of the ridge which is undercut relative to the path of displacement (2).

In this example, providing retention by engaging the distal undercut of the canine may well look more pleasing than a clasp arm on the same tooth.

The choice of tilt for the final survey of the study cast will usually be a compromise as the requirements of different parts of the denture often conflict, e.g. the appearance of a maxillary anterior saddle will tend to take precedence over the optimum positioning of molar clasps and thus a posterior tilt would be selected for the final survey. It is of course possible to create more favourable undercuts on the molars by tooth preparation (Chapter 21).

155

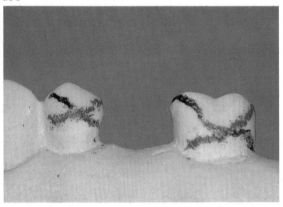

Final survey

155 If it is decided that the cast should be tilted, the analysing rod is exchanged for a marker different in colour from that used in the first survey, and the final survey is carried out. It will then usually be found that the teeth to be clasped have two separate survey lines which cross each other. In order to obtain optimum retention it is necessary to understand how to position the clasps correctly in relation to the two survey lines.

The aims for optimum retention should be to provide:

1 resistance along the path of displacement,
2 resistance along the path of withdrawal.

The former can be achieved by the use of guide surfaces or clasps while the latter is provided by clasps alone. The various ways of achieving these aims are illustrated in **156** to **159**. In each case the red survey line has been produced with the cast tilted and is relative to the path of insertion and withdrawal while the green survey line has been produced with the cast horizontal and is relative to the path of displacement.

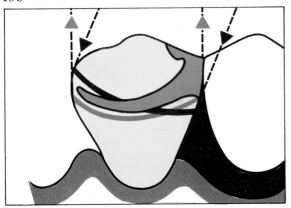

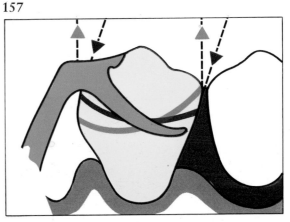

156 When guide surfaces are used to provide resistance to displacement of the denture in an occlusal direction, the retentive portion of the clasp needs only to resist movement along the path of withdrawal and therefore can be positioned solely with reference to the red survey line.

When the denture does not contact guide surfaces on the clasped tooth the clasp will have to resist movement of the denture along both the path of withdrawal and the path of displacement. The clasp will thus need to be positioned in the correct depth of undercut relative to both survey lines, so that it will

157 It does not matter if, as in this example, the clasp engages too deep an undercut relative to the path of displacement. Movement of the denture in an occlusal direction is prevented by contact with the guide surface, therefore permanent deformation of the clasp will not occur.

provide the necessary retention without being permanently deformed either by insertion and removal of the denture along the planned path or by inadvertent displacement of the denture during function. Ways of achieving this are shown in **158** and **159**.

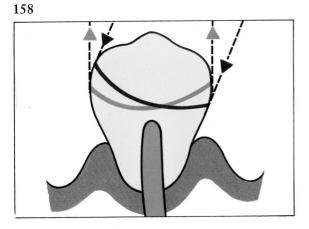

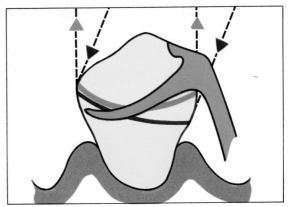

158 A gingivally approaching clasp positioned at the cross-over point of the survey lines resists movement along both the path of withdrawal and the path of displacement without being permanently deformed by movement along either path.

159 If the survey lines converge mesially or distally, the tip of an occlusally approaching clasp can engage the common area of undercut to provide resistance to movement along both paths.

If the cast has been tilted for the final survey, the degree of tilt must be recorded so that the position of the cast can be reproduced in the laboratory.

There are two methods of recording the degree of tilt:

160

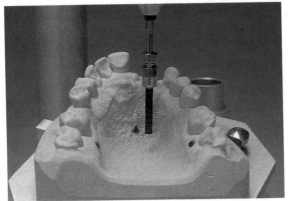

160 Using the tripod method, the vertical arm of the surveyor is locked at a height which allows the tip of the marker to contact the palatal surface of the ridge in the molar and incisal regions. Three points are marked with the graphite marker, one on each side posteriorly and one anteriorly. The points will then be ringed with a pencil so that they are clearly visible.

161

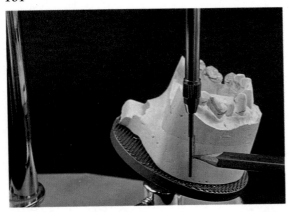

161 Alternatively, the analysing rod is placed against one side of the base of the cast and a line drawn on the cast parallel to the rod. This is repeated on the other side and at the back of the cast so that there are three widely spaced lines parallel to the path of insertion.

Summary of the clinical objectives of surveying

Surveying is undertaken to obtain information which will allow decisions to be made concerning the following:

1 The optimum path of insertion of the denture.
   The choice of a path of insertion will be influenced by:
   (a) the need to utilise guiding surfaces to achieve a pleasing appearance,
   (b) the need to avoid interference by the teeth or ridges with correct positioning of denture components,
   (c) the need to utilise guide surfaces for retention.

2 The design, material and position of clasps.

Decisions on these aspects of clasps can be arrived at from measurement of the horizontal extent of undercut on abutment teeth and the identification of sites on the teeth to provide reciprocation either from guiding surfaces or from cross-arch reciprocation (Chapter 12).

9 Saddles

The saddle is that part of a partial denture which rests on and covers the alveolar ridge and which includes the artificial teeth and gumwork. It is naturally regarded by the patient as the most important component because it imparts both appearance and function to the denture. The clinician's major concerns are centred on:

The design of the occlusal surface
The base extension
The design of the polished surface
The material for the impression surface
The junction between saddle and abutment tooth

The design of the occlusal surface

It is fundamentally important to position the artificial teeth in such a way that even occlusal contact in the intercuspal position is achieved and occlusal balance is created where appropriate.

162 The width of the posterior artificial teeth may well play an important part in the success of a lower partial denture especially if a free-end saddle is present. It has been shown that the reduction in area of the occlusal table, by using narrow posterior teeth or reducing the length of the table by omitting teeth, will reduce the force to the underlying tissues during mastication by making penetration of the food bolus easier. This principle is illustrated by the artificial teeth replacing 35 and 36 and is in contrast to the teeth replacing 45, 46 and 47. A further advantage in reducing the buccolingual width of the teeth is the increase in space made for the tongue which may well have spread laterally following extraction of the natural teeth. Were the space to be unduly restricted, the tongue would tend to move the denture during normal function.

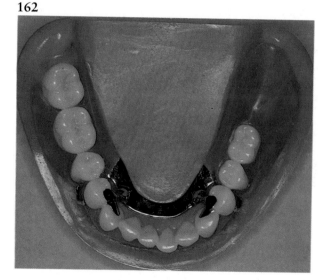
162

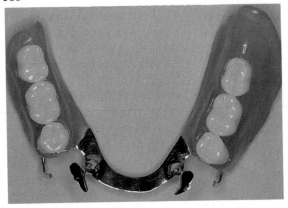

The base extension

163 When some, or all, of the support for a saddle is gained from the mucosa and underlying bone, the most important consideration is to ensure that the maximum possible area is covered by the base in order to distribute functional forces as widely as possible. This point is of particular relevance in the case of the free-end saddle denture where much of the force inevitably must be transmitted through the mucosa of the saddle area.

For this reason the base of the lower free-end saddle should be extended on to the retromolar pads and into the full functional depth of the buccal and lingual sulci, as in the saddle replacing 35, 36 and 37, so that the maximum area of bone, including the buccal shelf, is load-bearing. If coverage is reduced, as in the other saddle, both retention and stability will suffer and the stresses will be increased, thus putting the underlying bone at risk. When a saddle is fully tooth-supported, maximum extension of the base is not required for load distribution and it may therefore be reduced.

164a

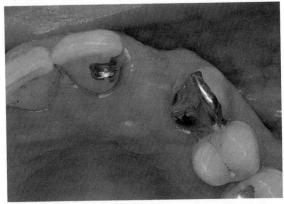

164b

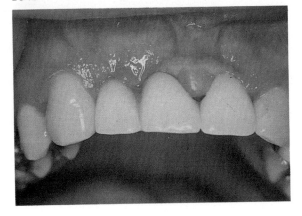

164a and **164b** The base extension of a small tooth-supported saddle at the front of the mouth will often be governed by aesthetic requirements. In (a) there has been very little resorption of the ridge and thus the artificial tooth will look best if fitted directly against the mucosa without any labial flange. However, the same design in (b) is quite inappropriate because there has been considerable resorption, making it impossible to create a good appearance without using a labial flange for 12, 11 and 21.

Design of the polished surface

165 The polished surface of the denture saddle is that surface which lies between the denture border and the occlusal surface, indicated by the black shading. The muscles of the lips, cheeks and tongue press against this surface. If the saddle is shaped correctly, the muscular forces will enhance retention and stability. But if the shape is incorrect the activity of the musculature will tend to displace the denture.

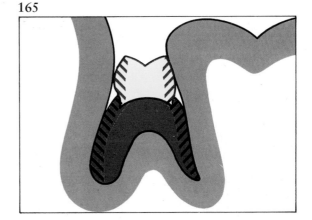

166 There is a space between tongue and cheeks where the opposing muscular forces are in balance. This space is known as the neutral zone or zone of minimal conflict. The concept of placing the denture within muscle balance is particularly important when designing free-end saddles because less mechanical retention is possible and thus greater reliance must be placed on muscle control.

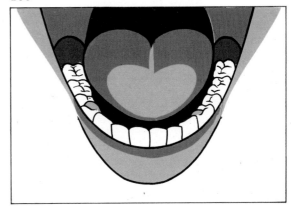

167 The free-end saddle replacing 45, 46 and 47 has been incorrectly shaped. The molars are placed lingually and interfere with the tongue space. Every time the tongue moves it lifts the denture.

If the teeth are moved buccally as in the case of 35, 36 and 37, the tongue is provided with sufficient space and its muscular force will now play a positive role in stabilising the denture.

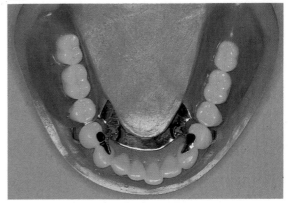

The mesial and distal margins of the base should be thinned so that any step between flanges and mucosa is minimised. This will reduce the tendency for food to lodge at this junction, will improve tolerance and, towards the front of the mouth, can make a major contribution to the appearance (**448** and **449**).

Material for the impression surface

The surface of the saddle in contact with the mucosa may be constructed in either metal or acrylic resin. An acrylic surface can be modified and added to with ease, a particular advantage where continuing bone resorption is expected as in the case of the free-end saddle.

168

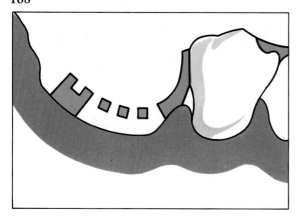

168 In cases where the clinician has decided on an acrylic impression surface, the material is retained on the metal framework via a spaced meshwork which has been constructed to lie above the mucosal surface. A small 'stop' of metal which contacts the surface of the cast in the free-end edentulous areas may be included. This 'stop' is a valuable reference point when the fit of the framework is checked both on the cast and in the mouth. Lack of contact between the 'stop' and the mucosa should be eliminated at the earliest possible stage by the altered cast technique (Chapter 25).

169

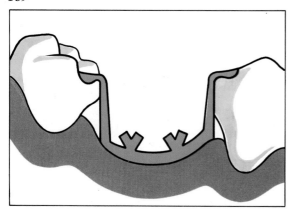

169 Where the impression surface is made in metal, more space is available for the artificial teeth. This method is thus of particular value in tooth-borne saddles where vertical space has been restricted by overerupted teeth.

170

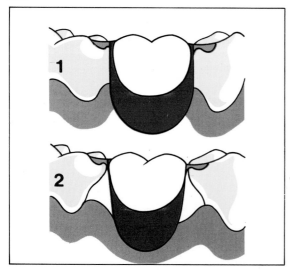

Junction between saddle and abutment tooth

170 Controversy exists in the dental literature as to whether there should be widespread contact between the saddle and abutment tooth, the *closed design* in (1), or whether the contact should be restricted to a small area close to the occlusal surface with generous clearance created at the gingival margin, the so-called *open design* as in (2). Although there appears to be no difference in the rate of plaque formation associated with the two designs, a higher temperature of the gingival tissues has been recorded when a closed design has been used. This result may be due to a change in quality of the bacterial plaque causing increased irritation of the gingival tissues.

171 An advantage of the closed design is that the guide-surface philosophy can be adopted (**137** and **138**), although it should be remembered that effective guide surfaces can be provided with an open design if the clinical crowns are of sufficient length. Furthermore, it will be appreciated that guide surfaces can be created on the lingual or palatal surfaces of teeth and that reciprocating elements can be positioned to contact these surfaces (**240** to **242**).

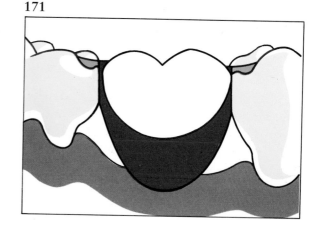

As with so many judgements, the choice of design for a particular patient depends on a number of factors. For example, if the prospect for effective retention using conventional clasp arms is poor, it may be advisable to create guide surfaces and use a closed design.

On the other hand, if plaque control is suspect, the decision may swing towards the open design in order to reduce gingival margin coverage to a minimum. A closed design may be required for an anterior saddle in order to produce a good appearance.

172a

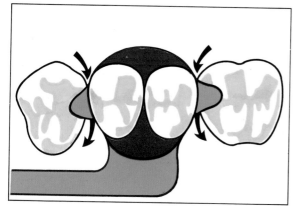

172b

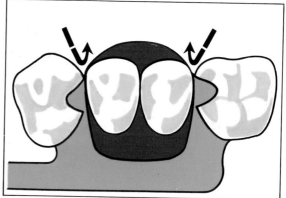

172a and **172b** It should be appreciated that the full benefits of the open design will be realised only if care is taken with the shaping of the flanges and the underlying framework. In (**a**) the denture has been so constructed that the advantages of the 'open' design are fully realised. In contrast, (**b**) shows a connector which has closed off one side of the interdental spaces.

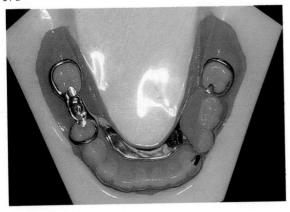

173 If appearance is not a problem, the philosophy of an 'open' design can be taken a stage further by constructing a so-called 'cleansable' pontic as at 46. The underside of the pontic is highly polished.

Finally, in this chapter, mention should be made of a design of saddle which contacts the maximum possible area – the two-part or sectional denture. This appliance is described in **227**.

10 Support

174a to **174c** Support may be defined as resistance to vertical force directed towards the mucosa. During function, this force is transmitted through the saddles of the partial denture and is ultimately resisted by the bone. If the denture rests solely on the mucoperiosteum, the force is transmitted via that tissue and the denture is termed 'mucosa-borne' (**a**). If the denture is supported on adjacent teeth by components such as occlusal rests, the force is transmitted to the bone via teeth and periodontal ligaments and the denture is described as 'tooth-borne' (**b**). When a saddle has an abutment tooth at one end only (a free-end saddle), the denture can at best be 'tooth/mucosa-borne' (**c**). The benefits of tooth-borne and the potential dangers of mucosa-borne dentures have been indicated in **21** and **22**.

174a

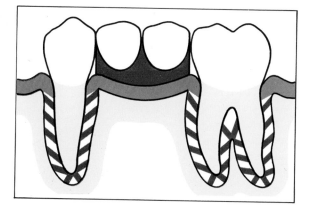

174b

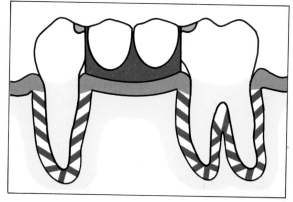

174c

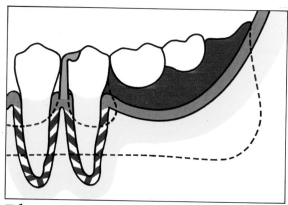

Planning support

When planning the denture design, a conscious decision must be made on the type of support most appropriate for the particular case. This decision is based on an assessment of:

1 the root area of the abutment teeth,
2 the extent of the saddles,
3 the expected force on the saddles.

175

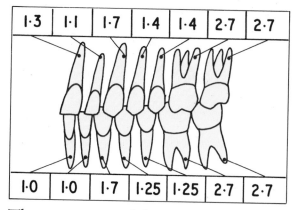

The root area of the abutment teeth

175 The area of root available to accept vertical force is governed by the type of tooth and by its periodontal health. The tooth with the least root area is the lower incisor. If this tooth is given unit value, the ratios of the root areas of the other teeth are as shown in this figure.

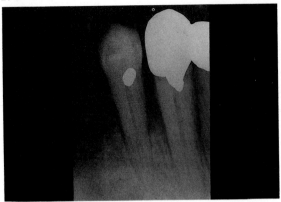

176 If the periodontal ligament has been partly destroyed by periodontal disease the full support potential of that tooth cannot be realised. It will also be appreciated that periodontal disease first attacks the widest part of the root and thus its greatest area. In this example the available root area has been reduced by approximately two-thirds.

177

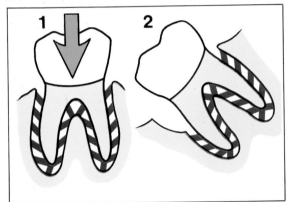

177 Most of the vertical force will be transmitted by the oblique fibres of the periodontal ligament (1). This large group of fibres will not function as effectively if the tooth is tilted (2). Commonly, the lower molar teeth are tilted mesially. There is often more bone resorbed on the mesial side of the tooth – a factor which aggravates the situation.

178

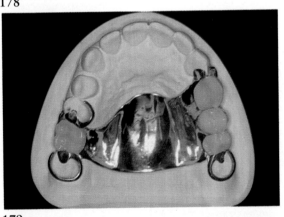

Extent of saddles

178 The smaller the saddle, the lower the functional forces. In this example the forces transmitted through the saddles can be borne safely by the abutment teeth.

179

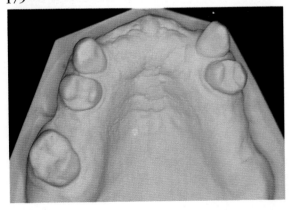

179 In the restoration of these extensive saddles the tooth support offered by the remaining teeth must be augmented by mucosal support derived from extensive palatal coverage.

180 It is of course possible to gain support from more than one tooth. In this instance, occlusal rests have been placed on both premolars so that the forces from the free-end saddle are distributed widely. However, the occlusal rest on the first premolar will share the supportive function only if there is minimal downward movement of the saddle when a vertical load is applied. A larger movement will cause the rest to rotate away from the tooth.

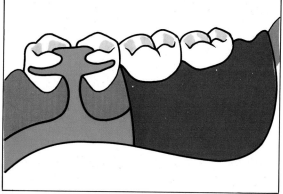

The expected force on the saddles

181 We have already mentioned that the magnitude of force will increase as the artificial occlusal surface increases in area. The magnitude can also be expected to vary with the nature of the opposing dentition. Studies have shown that the functional force created by an opposing denture will be less than that arising from several natural teeth.

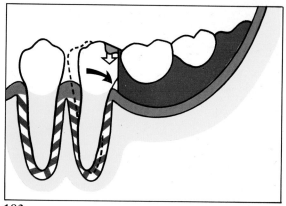

Tooth support for free-end saddles

182 The support of free-end saddles, especially in the mandible, is a particular problem and the optimum site for a rest is controversial. One view is that placing a distal rest on the abutment tooth encourages distal tipping of that tooth.

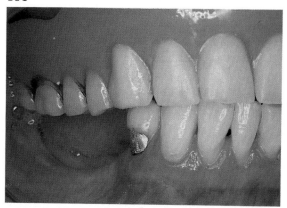

183 On the other hand, the placement of a mesial rest would tend to tip the abutment tooth mesially. Such movement would be resisted by contact with the adjacent tooth.

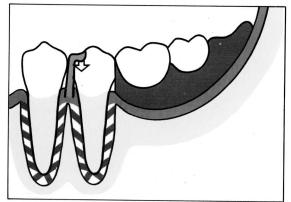

184

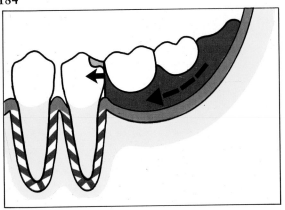

184 However, *in vitro* and *in vivo* studies have shown that the movement of the abutment tooth is usually in a mesial direction even when a distal rest is used. This may be due in part to the influence of the slope of the ridge on denture movement when the saddle is loaded. For this reason the argument for a mesial rest for free-end saddles is not as clear-cut as was once thought. However, the results of photoelastic studies, indicating more favourable stress distribution over the bone supporting the abutment tooth and the bone in the edentulous area, continue to justify the use of a mesial rest wherever possible.

In concluding this general discussion on principles of support, two final points should be made.

First, where the outlook of the patient and the state of the mouth indicate that a partial denture is expected to have a long life, every effort should be made to secure tooth support. Second, a mucosa-borne denture is likely to be more successful in the upper jaw than in the lower jaw as palatal coverage ensures more effective support. More often than not, a mucosa-borne denture in the lower jaw causes tissue damage.

The remainder of this section will now be devoted to a more detailed consideration of components used to obtain tooth support.

185

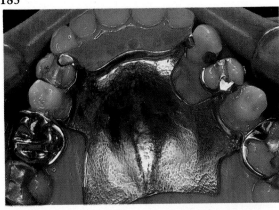

185 A denture may be supported on premolars or molars by occlusal rests and on upper canines by cingulum rests as on 23.

186

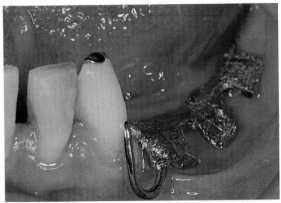

186 Support may be gained from lower canines by incisal rests.

Upper and lower canines require these different designs because the lower usually does not possess a sufficiently well developed cingulum in which a rest seat can be prepared.

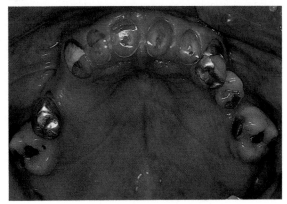

187 A rather different approach to support is offered by overdenture abutment teeth. These anterior teeth, already severely worn, have been shaped to create dome-shaped preparations. When they are covered by a partial denture the vertical force will be directed down the long axes of the teeth.

Additional functions of rests

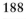

1 Distribution of horizontal force
2 Maintaining components in their correct position
3 Protecting the denture/abutment tooth junction
4 Providing indirect retention
5 Reciprocation
6 Preventing overeruption
7 Improving occlusal contact

Distribution of horizontal force

188 In addition to the vitally important function of transferring vertical forces through the root of the tooth and thence to the alveolar bone, certain shapes of rest will transfer some of the horizontal functional force; this is known as the bracing function (Chapter 12).

For example, the portion of the cingulum rest on the canine which lies against the side of the tooth will transmit some horizontal force to the tooth. Whether or not this is appropriate for a particular tooth depends upon the periodontal support of that tooth.

188

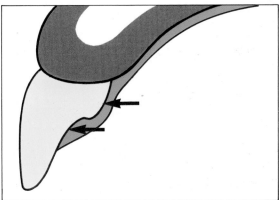

189

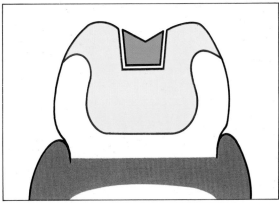

189 An occlusal rest which has been placed in a saucer-shaped rest seat will transmit less horizontal force to the tooth than will a rest placed in a box-shaped rest seat prepared in a cast gold restoration. This box-shaped preparation, if sufficiently deep, will also provide guide-surfaces to control the path of insertion of the denture. The amount of horizontal force which it is permissible to transmit to a tooth is dependent upon its periodontal health. Needless to say, this latter method can be employed only on a tooth which has sufficient root area for support and whose periodontal condition is perfectly healthy. In reality the technique can be used on few occasions.

Maintaining components in their correct position

If a partial denture is fully supported on natural teeth it will not sink into the underlying tissues and therefore the various components will be held in the position they were originally designed to occupy.

190

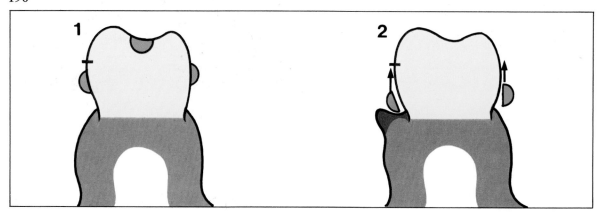

190 (1) If the retentive clasp still maintains its original position relative to the maximum bulbosity of the tooth, it will act immediately the denture is displaced occlusally. (2) If through lack of support, the denture has sunk into the supporting tissues and the clasp has retreated cervically, the denture will move some distance before the retentive tip commences to resist the displacement. Thus it can be seen that the rest improves the efficiency of a retentive clasp as well as keeping it well clear of the gingival margin, thus avoiding trauma to the mucosa.

191

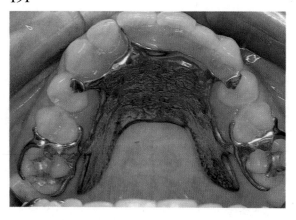

Protecting the denture/abutment tooth junction

191 The occlusal rest may provide an effective roof to the space between saddle and abutment tooth as in this instance between 23 and 24. Although it will not prevent ingress of material from the buccal and lingual aspects, it will protect the gingival tissues from food being forcibly pushed down between denture and tooth by the power strokes of mastication.

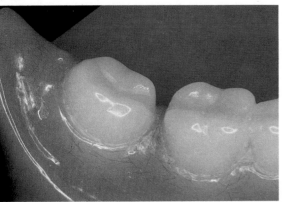

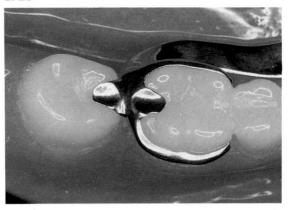

192a and **192b** Occlusal rests can also be used to bridge a gap between teeth, thus again providing an effective roof over the vulnerable interdental area.

Providing indirect retention

This concept is discussed fully in Chapter 13. A rest is one of the components which is capable of providing indirect retention.

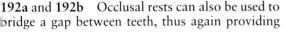

Reciprocation

This principle is described in Chapter 12. A rest placed in a box-shaped preparation in a molar or premolar tooth can provide effective reciprocation for a retentive clasp, as can a cingulum rest for a retentive clasp on the labial surface of a canine.

Preventing overeruption

The position of a tooth is best maintained by contact of an opposing tooth, be it natural or artificial. In the absence of an opposing tooth, a well-retained occlusal rest is able to prevent over-eruption.

Improving occlusal contact

193 On occasions, the support may be provided by the more widespread coverage of an onlay. This variation may be chosen when there is a need to improve the occlusal contact of the teeth.

193

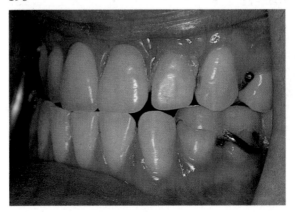

11 Retention

194

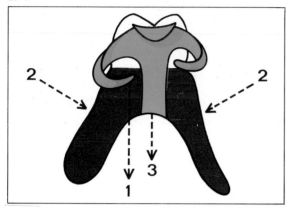

194 Retention of a partial denture can be achieved by using *mechanical means* (1) such as clasps which engage undercuts on the tooth surface, by harnessing the patient's *muscular control* (2) acting through the polished surface of the denture, and by using the inherent *physical forces* (3) which arise from coverage of the mucosa by the denture. Whether reliance is placed on all or mainly on one of these methods depends on clinical circumstances. Retention by mechanical means can also be obtained by selecting a path of insertion which permits rigid components to enter undercut areas on teeth or on ridges (**151** and **154**).

195

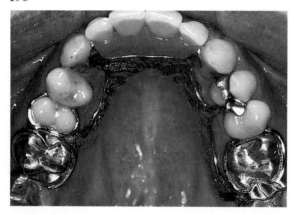

195 In this particular case there are sufficient teeth with suitable undercut areas to allow the partial denture to be retained by clasps. Successful clasp retention allows the palatal coverage to be reduced to a minimum. Not only is this limited coverage appreciated by the patient but it reduces the risk of damage to the oral tissues.

196

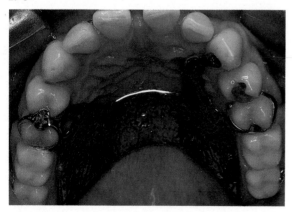

196 In contrast to the previous case, this patient's remaining teeth offer less opportunity for clasp retention. It is necessary, therefore, to cover more of the palate in order to harness the physical forces of retention.

197 Muscular control is of particular importance for the success of an extensive lower bilateral free-end saddle denture. Although this denture achieves some retention from clasps its success will depend particularly on the muscles of the tongue and cheeks acting on the correctly designed polished surfaces of the saddles.

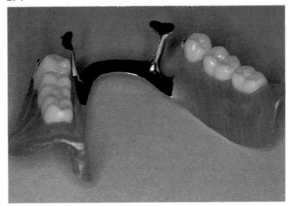

As will be seen later in this section, there are circumstances where there is a tendency for retentive clasps to lose some of their efficiency with the passage of time. Thus, in the long term, successful retention may become more dependent upon the physical forces and muscular control. However, it is generally accepted that retentive clasps are particularly beneficial during the early stages of denture-wearing as they ensure effective mechanical retention while the patient learns the appropriate muscular skills which will either augment or replace the contribution of the clasps.

The remainder of this section is devoted to a consideration of components which provide mechanical retention, namely clasps, precision attachments and other devices.

Clasps

198 Although many designs of retentive clasps have been described, they can be considered in one of two broad categories: the occlusally approaching clasp on 27 and the gingivally approaching clasp on 23.

— occlusally > approaching
— gingival

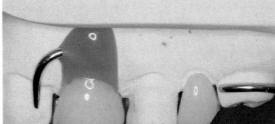

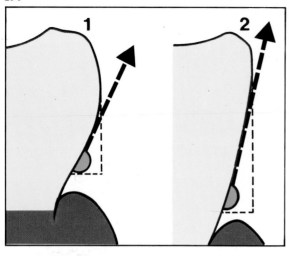

199 Whatever type of clasp is used, a denture will be retained successfully only as long as the force required to flex the clasps over the maximum bulbosities of the teeth is greater than the force which is attempting to dislodge the denture. The retentive force is dictated by tooth shape and by clasp design.

It is immediately obvious that the retentive force of a clasp is directly related to the depth of horizontal undercut engaged. It is perhaps less apparent that the force is also related to the steepness of the undercut. Clasps (1) and (2) are positioned in the same horizontal undercut (0.25 mm). However, clasp (1) must climb over a steeper 'hill' before it escapes over the maximum bulbosity of the tooth. Thus, the retention it offers is greater than that of clasp (2).

200 The flexibility of a retentive clasp is dependent upon its design. Round section and half-round section clasps flex easily in the horizontal plane but the half-round clasp is more resistant to movement in the vertical plane. The longer the arm, the more flexible will be the clasp. Thus the clasp on a molar will be more flexible than that on a premolar. Thickness has a profound effect on flexibility. If the thickness is reduced by half, the flexibility is increased by a factor of eight.

201 Flexibility is also dependent upon the alloy used to construct the clasp. The most commonly used alloy, cobalt chromium, has a value for modulus of elasticity (stiffness) indicated by the steepness of the first part of the solid black curve, which is twice that of gold (the red dotted curve). Thus, under identical conditions the force required to deflect the cobalt chromium clasp over the bulbosity of the tooth will be twice that of a gold clasp.

Of particular importance is the proportional limit of the alloy indicated by the solid circles on the curves. If a clasp is stressed beyond the proportional limit it will be distorted permanently. Hard gold and cobalt chromium have similar proportional limits. Hardened stainless steel wire (blue broken curve) has a much higher value.

It will be appreciated that the factors mentioned above interact with each other. Thus the choice of an appropriate clasp which will retain a denture satisfactorily and yet not stress the tooth unduly or be distorted perman-ently during service might appear to be some-what bewildering. In this Atlas we feel it is appropriate to offer the following clinical guidelines which have been shown to work in practice.

202a and **202b** As shown in (**a**), a cobalt chromium clasp arm, approximately 15 mm long, should be placed in a horizontal undercut of 0.25 mm. If the undercut is less the retention will be inadequate. If it is greater, the clasp arm will be distorted because the proportional limit is likely to be exceeded. A cobalt chromium occlusally approaching clasp engaging the same amount of undercut on a premolar tooth (**b**) is likely to distort during function because it is too short. In such a situation one can lengthen the clasp arm by using a gingivally approaching design. Whether this choice is appropriate depends on certain clinical factors which will be highlighted later in this chapter. Alternatively, an alloy with a lower modulus of elasticity but similar proportional limit, such as a platinum–gold–palladium wire, can be used.

Yet another possibility is to use a material with a higher proportional limit but similar modulus; wrought stainless steel or cobalt chromium (Wiptam) wires are suitable.

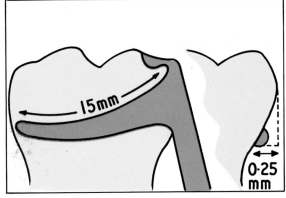

202a

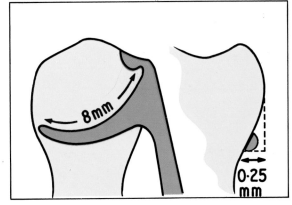

202b

203 Whether a gold or stainless steel clasp arm can be provided depends on the configuration of the denture. In this example the gold clasps can be held securely within the acrylic of the saddles.

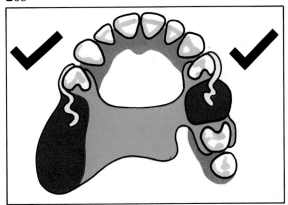

203

204 If a gold clasp were to be provided for 24, its only means of attachment to the remainder of the denture would be by soldering it to the cobalt chromium framework. Such a union is relatively weak and thus is prone to fracture during use.

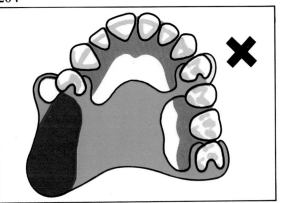

204

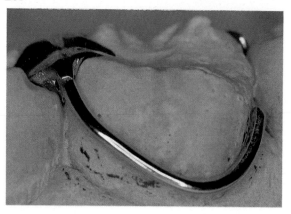

205 A cobalt chromium 'Wiptam' round wire clasp can be attached to the framework using a 'cast-on' technique.

Where it is necessary to add clasp retention to an acrylic transitional denture, stainless steel wire is a relatively inexpensive solution to the problem. Wire of 0.75 mm diameter is appropriate for premolar teeth while 1 mm diameter wire is suitable for molar teeth.

Two final points are worth making before we leave the subject of clasp construction and progress to further consideration of design and clinical use. First, the efficiency of a retentive clasp is also dictated by the support of the denture (**190**) and by reciprocation (**240** and **241**). Second, it is comforting to know that the variables of clasp construction have been neatly simplified by manufacturers who produce preformed wax patterns whose shapes have been designed according to type of tooth and alloy that is to be used.

Comparison of occlusally and gingivally approaching clasps

Retention

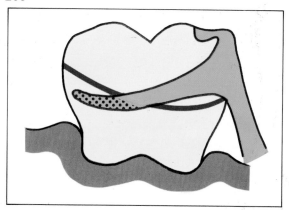

206 Only the terminal third of an occlusally approaching clasp (stippled section) should cross the survey line and enter the undercut area. If, in error, too much of the clasp arm engages the undercut, the high force required to pull it over the maximum bulbosity will put a considerable strain on the fibres of the periodontal ligament and is likely to exceed the proportional limit of the alloy, thus distorting the clasp.

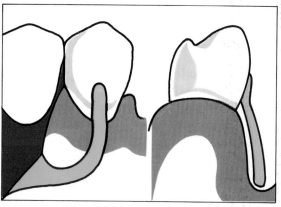

207 A gingivally approaching clasp contacts the tooth surface only at its tip. The remainder of the clasp arm is free of contact with the mucosa of the sulcus and the gingival margin. The length of the arm gives the clasp more flexibility than the occlusally approaching clasp – a positive advantage when it is necessary to clasp a premolar tooth or a tooth whose periodontal attachment has been reduced by periodontal disease.

Bracing (Chapter 12)

208 As the occlusally approaching clasp is more rigid and as more of it (stippled section) is in contact with the tooth surface above the survey line, it is capable of transmitting more horizontal force to the tooth. Whether such a measure is appropriate depends upon the health of the periodontal tissues.

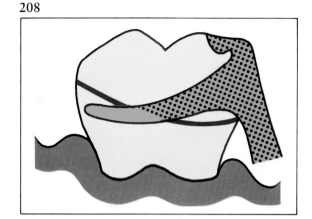

209

Appearance

209 Either type of clasp can detract from appearance when placed on a tooth which is towards the front of the mouth. The gingivally approaching clasp has more potential for being hidden in the distobuccal aspect of a tooth provided that there is a suitable undercut area for the clasp.

Hygiene

The gingivally approaching clasp can be criticised on the grounds that it crosses a gingival margin. There does not appear to be any evidence to indicate that one clasp encourages more plaque than the other. However, it is not unreasonable to assume that, if good oral hygiene is not practised by the patient, the gingivally approaching clasp will pose a greater threat to periodontal health.

Mention should also be made of the gingivally approaching clasp increasing the risk of root caries. It should be remembered that this lesion is strongly associated with gingival recession, which itself is age-related.

Factors governing the choice of retentive clasp

The choice of retentive clasp on an individual tooth depends upon:

1 the position of the undercut,
2 the health of the periodontal ligament,
3 the shape of the sulcus,
4 the length of clasp,
5 appearance.

As we have already discussed the significance of length of clasp and appearance, particular attention will be focused on the first three factors.

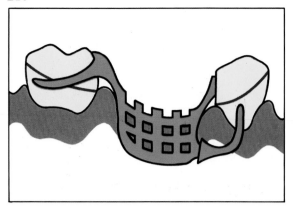

The position of the undercut

210 The diagonal survey lines on the molar and premolar teeth shown here ensure that there is a larger undercut on that part of the tooth which is *furthest* away from the saddle area. Typical designs of retentive clasp are the occlusally approaching clasp on the molar and the gingivally approaching 'I' bar on the premolar tooth.

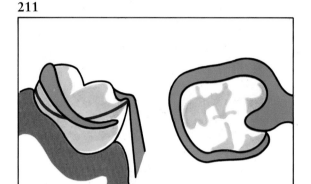

211 The orientation of the diagonal survey line on this molar creates the larger undercut area *nearer* to the saddle. The design of occlusally approaching clasp used on the molar in **210** would be quite inappropriate because it would prove difficult to keep the non-retentive two-thirds of the clasp out of the undercut whilst, at the same time, offering very little for the retentive portion. An alternative design is the 'ring' clasp which commences on the opposite side of the tooth and attacks the diagonal survey line from a more appropriate direction. An 'I' bar would be suitable for a premolar tooth with a survey line of similar orientation.

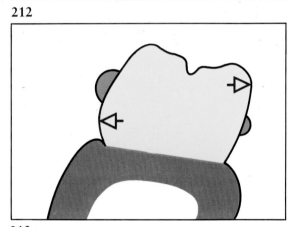

212 A low survey line (on the left side of the tooth) is present because the tooth is tilted; thus there is a high survey line on the other side of the tooth. Again, a 'ring' clasp is a solution to the problem: the bracing portion of the clasp is on the left side of the tooth and the retentive portion on the right side.

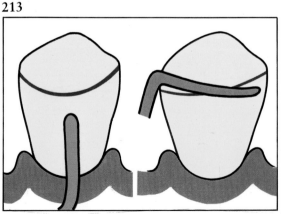

213 A high survey line poses particular difficulties on a premolar tooth. If it is not appropriate or practical to lower the survey line by altering the crown shape, it may be possible to position a flexible gingivally approaching clasp higher up the crown or, if an occlusally approaching clasp is unavoidable, to use a more flexible platinum–gold–palladium wrought wire clasp.

The health of the periodontal ligament

If a retentive clasp is placed on a tooth, it is inevitable that extra force will be transmitted to the supporting tissues of that tooth. Whether or not these tissues are able to absorb the extra force without suffering damage depends upon their health, the area of attachment and the magnitude of the force.

214 This canine tooth has already lost approximately half its periodontal attachment as a result of previous periodontal disease. Although the disease process has been arrested, there is every likelihood that further damage will occur if a relatively inflexible retentive clasp system, such as a cobalt chromium occlusally approaching clasp, is provided. If it is considered essential to rely on mechanical retention, a reasonable solution is to prescribe a more flexible gingivally approaching clasp such as an 'I' bar.

214

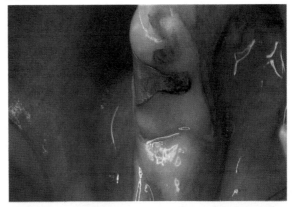

The shape of the sulcus

215 If a gingivally approaching clasp is envisaged, the shape of the sulcus must be checked carefully to ensure that there are no anatomical obstacles. In this example the prominent fraenal attachment would be traumatised by a gingivally approaching clasp of correct proportions. If there is no reasonable alternative to this clasp, and mechanical retention is thought to be essential, serious consideration must be given to surgical excision of the fraenal attachments.

215

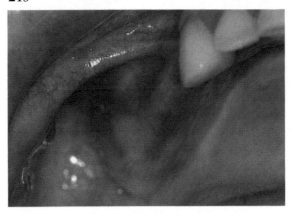

216 If there is an undercut in the sulcus, the arm of a gingivally approaching clasp must lie away from the mucosa to allow the denture to be inserted and removed. If the undercut is deep, the space between clasp arm and mucosa may be so great that it would be an intolerable nuisance to the patient.

216

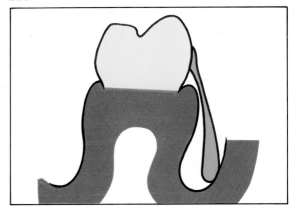

The RPI system

So far we have described a number of different clasps and have made the point that inflexible clasp systems can be detrimental to the tooth-supporting tissues. Nowhere is this more critical than at the free-end saddle where mechanical retention has frequently to be gained on premolar teeth, and where every endeavour should be made to distribute the masticatory loads between the tissues of the edentulous area and abutment teeth according to their ability to resist them.

217

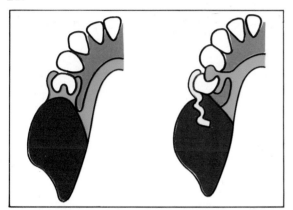

217 A number of photoelastic studies have shown that, if the occlusal rest is placed on the distal aspect of the abutment tooth and the clasp is occlusally approaching (left), more load is placed on the abutment tooth and the remainder is transmitted to the tissues of the edentulous area more unevenly. More favourable loading occurs when the rest is placed on the mesial aspect of the tooth and a more flexible clasp design, such as a platinum–gold–palladium wrought wire, is used (right).

218

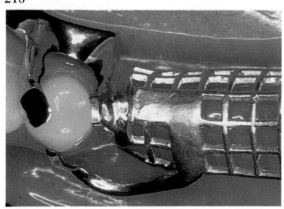

218 The above realisation led to the concept of the RPI system
R = mesial Rest
P = distal guiding Plate
I = I-shaped retentive clasp, commonly called an I bar.
The minor connector carrying the mesial rest contacts the mesiolingual surface of the abutment tooth and, together with the distal plate, acts as a reciprocal to the tip of the retentive clasp which is positioned on or anterior to the midpoint of the buccal surface of the tooth.

219

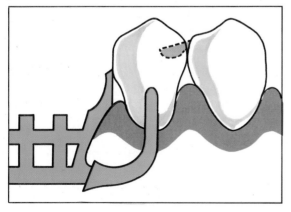

219 The guide plate moves down the guide surface which is prepared on the distal aspect of the tooth. When the denture is fully seated, the plate contacts the lower part of that surface.

220 As the saddle is pressed into the denture-bearing mucosa during function, the denture tends to rotate about a point close to the mesial rest. Both plate and I bar move in the direction indicated and are likely to disengage from the tooth surface. Neither of these components will therefore stress the abutment tooth unduly during their paths of movement, provided that the metal framework is carefully adjusted in the mouth to allow for this rotation.

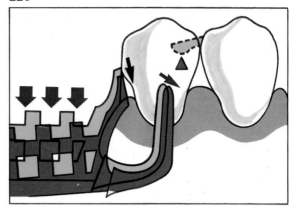

Precision attachments

A precision attachment is made up of two components, one of which is attached to the abutment tooth and the other housed in the denture. When the two matched parts are linked together they produce very positive retention. It is not the purpose of this Atlas to provide detailed information on precision attachments but rather to note their existence and refer the reader to texts which deal with this topic in an admirable manner.

221 The attachment on 46 is an example of the intracoronal type. A slot is incorporated within the substance of a crown and is engaged by a matching component on the removable section.

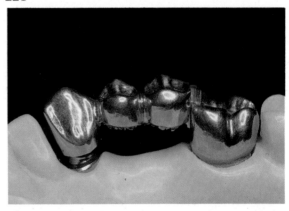

222 The extracoronal attachment, such as the Dalbo, is attached to the outside of the crown. The matched component held in the denture is designed to allow rotatory movement as the free-end saddle sinks into the denture-bearing mucosa, thus taking some of the stress off the abutment tooth.

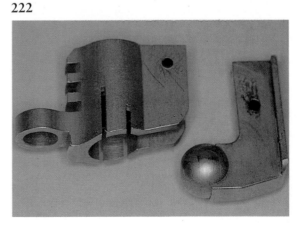

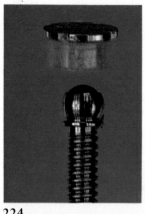
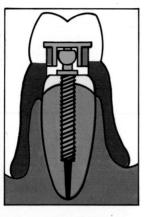

223 With the attachments, like the Kurer system, the stud is fixed to the root face of a root-filled tooth and a retainer held in the acrylic of the denture base snaps over the stud.

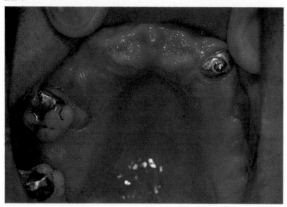

224 In this example the stud attachment affords positive retention in the anterior region for the extensive saddles.

The advantages of precision attachments include positive retention in the absence of clasp arms. Their use necessitates extensive preparation of the abutment teeth and an inevitable increase in cost of treatment. The more rigid attachments require the abutment teeth to have particularly healthy periodontal tissues. As the attachments tend to encourage the formation of plaque, the standard of oral hygiene must be immaculate. Maintenance of the denture may be complicated by wear of the attachments which may necessitate replacement of the component parts.

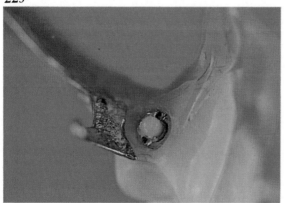

Other devices

225 The ZA anchor is an example of a spring-loaded attachment. The spring-loaded nipple engages an undercut on the surface of an abutment tooth adjacent to the saddle. It is used for retaining bounded saddles and is of particular value for upper canine or premolar teeth where a conventional clasp arm would detract from appearance.

226 In recent years there has been an increasing interest in the use of magnets. The modern alloys are powerful and retain their magnetism for a very long time. Each magnetic unit has a force of attraction in the region of 200–300 g, which is maximal as soon as the denture starts to move. This force of attraction imparts a degree of security to the denture without putting great demands on the periodontal tissues of the abutment teeth. In this example the bipolar magnet will be incorporated in the denture. The keeper is housed in a gold coping fitted to a root-filled tooth.

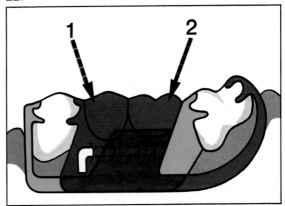

227 The two-part denture makes use of opposing undercuts. Both parts are inserted separately using different paths of insertion. In this figure the portion coloured blue is inserted first from a mesial direction to engage the mesial undercut on the molar. Then the magenta portion is inserted from a distal direction to engage the distal undercut on the premolar. Once the components are positioned they are locked together – in this instance with a bolt.

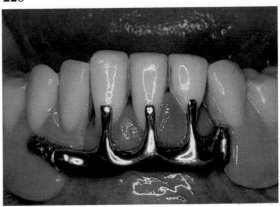

228 The Swing-lock denture has a hinged labial bar which has extensions into undercuts on the labial surfaces of the teeth. When the 'gate' is closed and locked into position, the denture is held securely by the 'gate' on the labial aspect and by the reciprocating components on the lingual aspects of the teeth. The denture can be particularly helpful where the remaining natural teeth offer very little undercut for conventional clasp retention. This patient, a trombone player, required a positively retained partial denture. The Swing-lock design allowed optimum use to be made of the incisors. As this type of denture covers a considerable amount of gingival margin, the standard of plaque control must be high.

There is an added advantage of the Swing-lock denture in that the 'gate' can carry a labial acrylic veneer. This veneer can be used to improve the appearance when a considerable amount of root surface has been exposed following periodontal surgery.

12 Bracing and reciprocation

Bracing

229

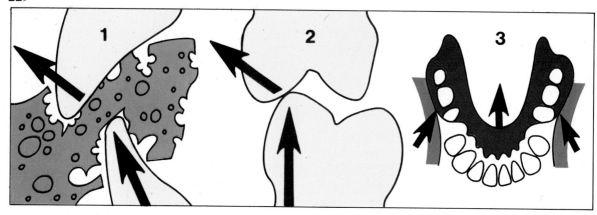

229 Horizontal forces are generated during function by occlusal contact (1 and 2) and by the oral musculature surrounding the denture (3).

These forces attempt to displace the denture in both *antero-posterior* and *lateral* directions.

230a

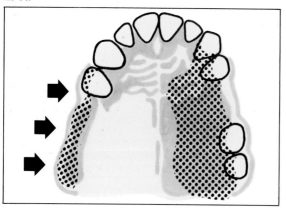

230b

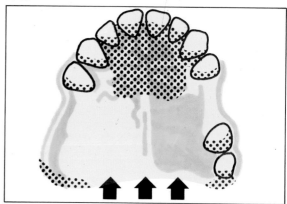

230a and **230b**   The horizontal forces are resisted by placing rigid components of the denture (bracing components) against suitable vertical surfaces on the teeth and residual ridges. Parts of a denture resting against the stippled areas will resist the forces whose directions are shown by the arrows. It is important to appreciate that bracing occurs only when the denture is *fully seated*.

231 The *lateral forces* in particular are capable of inflicting considerable damage on the periodontal tissues and alveolar bone in the edentulous areas. Thus they have to be carefully controlled. Bracing on teeth may be achieved by means of rigid portions of clasp arms (1) or plates (2). Bracing on the ridges and in the palate is obtained by means of major connectors and flanges (3).

A free-end saddle creates particular problems as it is capable of being displaced posteriorly and of rotating in the horizontal plane. Furthermore, the lateral force must be distributed widely so that tissue damage is avoided. The problems are more acute in the lower jaw.

231

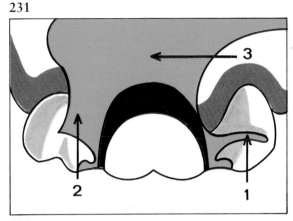

232 Those components of the partial denture coloured blue are capable of resisting lateral forces coming from the direction indicated by the arrows. Needless to say, lateral forces in the opposite direction will be resisted by the mirror images of these components.

232

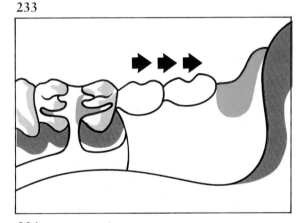

233 Posterior movement is prevented by coverage of the retromolar pads and by the minor connectors which contact the mesiolingual surfaces of the premolar teeth.

233

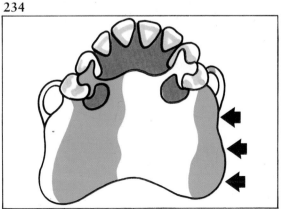

234 Effective distribution of the lateral force in the upper jaw is less of a problem as much of it can be transmitted to the bone of the palatal vault by extensive palatal coverage. Those components of the partial denture coloured blue are capable of resisting lateral forces coming from the direction indicated by the arrows.

234

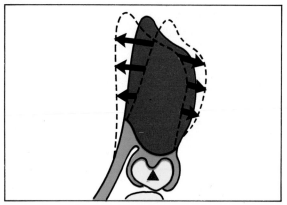

235 The posterior part of the free-end saddle is capable of rotating in the horizontal plane. If a long saddle is clasped rigidly to a single abutment tooth the rotatory movement can transmit considerable force to that tooth.

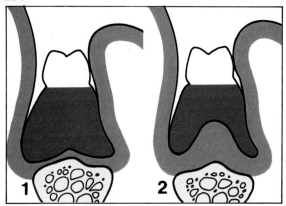

236 The flatter the ridge (1) or the more compressible the mucosa (2), the greater is the potential for movement. It should also be remembered that the close fit of a denture will deteriorate following resorption of the residual ridge. Once more the potential for rotatory movement is increased.

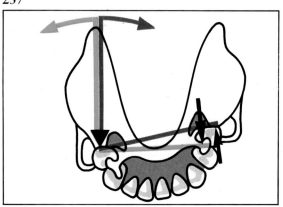

237 Rotation can be resisted effectively by this design which incorporates appropriately placed bracing elements and joins them with a rigid connector. Rotation of the right saddle in the direction of the blue arrow is resisted by the minor connector contacting the mesial surface of 35. Movement of the saddle in the direction of the red arrow will be resisted by the minor connector contacting the distal surface of the same tooth.

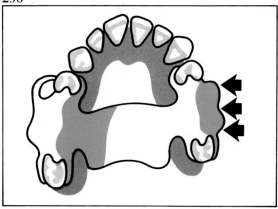

238 Rotation and anteroposterior movement of bounded saddles are resisted by contact of the saddles with the abutment teeth. It therefore remains to design bracing elements which will safely distribute the lateral forces acting on the denture. The bracing elements which oppose a lateral force indicated by the arrows are shown in this illustration.

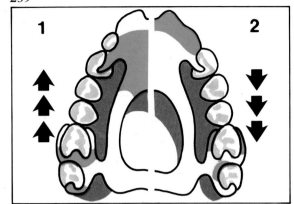

239 (1) Anterior displacement of an upper Kennedy Class IV denture can be resisted by elements of the framework contacting the disto-palatal surfaces of the teeth and, in some cases, by the connector covering the anterior slope of the palate. (2) Posterior displacement is prevented by the labial flange, by contact between the saddle and the mesial surface of 23, by contact of the minor connectors against the mesiopalatal surfaces of 27 and by the tips of clasp arms on 26.

240

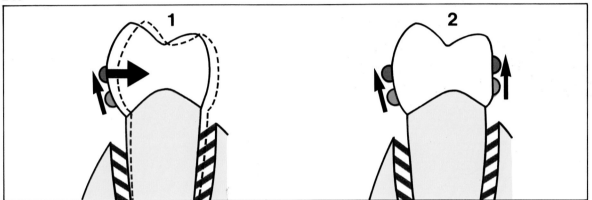

Reciprocation

240 The bracing element which is in contact with the side of the tooth opposite the retentive clasp can also play an important role in the effectiveness of the latter, and thus in the overall retention of the denture.

(1) A horizontally directed force is produced as a retentive arm is displaced in an occlusal direction over the bulbosity of a tooth. If the clasp arm is unopposed the tooth is displaced in the periodontal space and much of the retentive capability will be lost. (2) If the retentive clasp is opposed by a rigid component which maintains contact with the tooth as the retentive arm moves over the bulbosity of the tooth, displacement of the tooth is resisted, the retentive arm is forced to flex and thus the efficiency of the retentive element is increased. This principle is known as *reciprocation*. It is thus apparent that reciprocation is required as the denture is being displaced occlusally whilst the bracing function, as mentioned earlier, comes into play when the denture is fully seated.

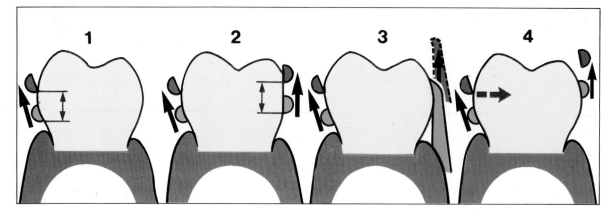

241 (1) A clasp is effective in retention over the distance from its position when the denture is fully seated to where it escapes over the bulbosity of the tooth. This vertical measurement may be termed the 'retention distance'. It will be appreciated that the reciprocal element on the other side of the tooth should be in continuous contact with the tooth surface as the retentive arm traverses the 'retention distance'. Effective reciprocation can be achieved either (2) by a clasp arm contacting a guide surface of similar height to the 'retention distance', or (3) by a plate making continuous contact with the tooth surface as the retentive arm moves through its 'retention distance'.

(4) If the reciprocating clasp is placed on a tooth without an adequate guide surface, it will lose contact with the tooth before the retentive arm has passed over the maximum bulbosity of the tooth and fail to provide effective reciprocation.

242

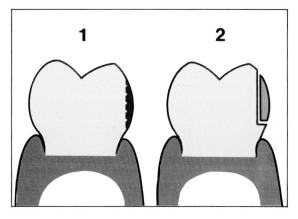

242 On rare occasions it may be possible to find a guide surface which occurs naturally on a tooth. More often it will be necessary to create a suitable surface (1) by minimal shaping of the enamel or (2) by building the appropriate surface into a cast metal restoration, always supposing that such an extensive restoration is justified on that particular tooth.

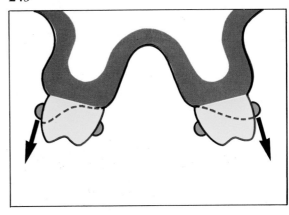

243 If the tooth surface on which the bracing arm is to be placed has the survey line at the level of the gingival margin, effective reciprocation on the same tooth may be impossible to achieve. In such circumstances one may use the principle of *cross-arch reciprocation*, where a retentive clasp on one side of the arch opposes a similar component on the other side. The retentive clasps can be placed either buccal/buccal (as in the illustration) or lingual/lingual. The disadvantage of this approach is that, as the bracing arms leave the tooth surfaces, the teeth will move in their sockets. This 'jiggling' action is potentially damaging to the supporting tissues.

13 Indirect retention

244

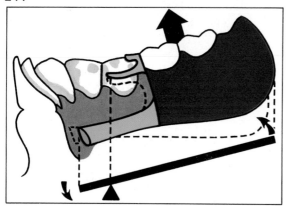

The principle of indirect retention may be explained by reference to the behaviour of a lower free-end saddle in function.

244 This denture has occlusal rests and clasps on the abutment teeth and the connector is a sublingual bar. When sticky foods displace the saddle in an occlusal direction the only resistance to the movement is provided by the tips of the retentive clasps engaging the undercuts on the abutment teeth. The saddle thus pivots about the clasp tip.

In the upper jaw this movement of the saddle away from the ridge may also be caused by gravity.

245

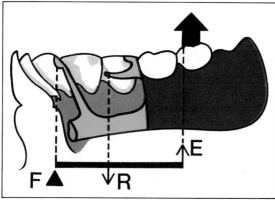

245 If the design is modified by placing a rest on an anterior tooth, this rest (indirect retainer) becomes the fulcrum of movement of the saddle in an occlusal direction causing the clasp to move up the tooth, engage the undercut, and thus resist the tendency for the denture to pivot.

F = FULCRUM – indirect retainer, a component which obtains support.

R = RESISTANCE – retention generated by the clasp.

E = EFFORT – displacing force, e.g. a bolus of sticky food.

It can thus be seen that to obtain indirect retention the clasp must always be placed *between* the saddle and the indirect retainer.

246

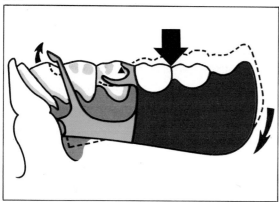

246 Indirect retainers do *not* prevent displacement *towards* the ridge. This movement is resisted by the occlusal rest on the abutment tooth and by full extension of the saddle to gain maximum support from the residual ridge. In addition, it may be necessary to compensate for the compressibility of the denture-bearing mucosa by using the altered cast impression technique (Chapter 25).

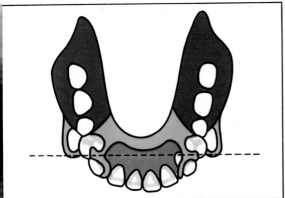

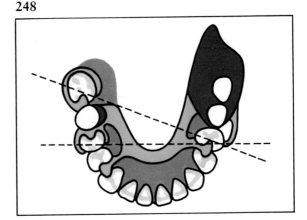

247 In order to understand the way in which indirect retainers are located it is necessary to consider the possible movement of the denture around an axis formed by the clasps. This clasp axis is defined as the line drawn between the retentive tips of a pair of clasps on opposite sides of the arch.

As the resistance to displacement in an occlusal direction of a saddle utilising indirect retention is provided by the clasps forming the clasp axis, the effectiveness of these clasps is of paramount importance in determining the amount of indirect retention obtained.

Mechanical disadvantage of the denture design

249 The clasp is always nearer to the indirect retainer (fulcrum) than is the displacing force. The clasp is therefore working at a mechanical disadvantage relative to the displacing force.

The partial denture design should strive to reduce the mechanical advantage of the displacing force by placing the clasp axis as near as possible to the saddle and by placing the indirect retainers as far as possible from the saddle.

248 Where there is more than one clasp axis, as in this unilateral free-end saddle denture, it is the clasps on the axis closer to the saddle in question which make the major contribution to indirect retention.

Other factors which influence the effectiveness of indirect retention are:
— the mechanical disadvantage of the denture design,
— the support of the indirect retainers.

249

effort arm

resistance arm

displacing force
E

F
indirect retainer

R
clasp

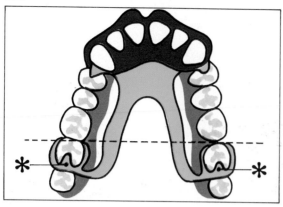

250 In this partial denture design the indirect retainers * are inefficient because they are placed too close to the clasp axis.

251

251 If the clasp axis is moved closer to the saddle and the indirect retainers * further away, the effectiveness of the indirect retention is improved.

252

Support for the indirect retainer

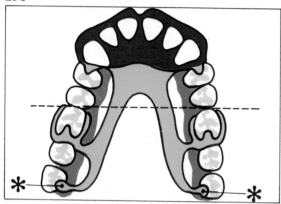

252 Tooth support is preferable to mucosal support because the compressibility of mucosa allows movement of the denture to occur.

If there is no alternative to mucosal support the indirect retainer should cover a sufficiently wide area to spread the load and avoid mucosal injury. This consideration effectively limits mucosally supported indirect retainers to the upper jaw where the load can be distributed over the hard palate (shaded area of the connector). However, this plan view is somewhat misleading as it suggests that the indirect retention achieved is more effective than it really is.

253

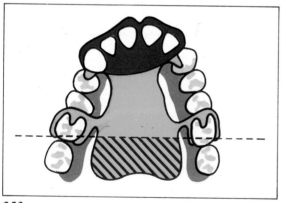

253 The side view (simplified) of the same design shows that, when the saddle is first displaced, mucosal compression beneath the indirect retainer allows the denture to rotate around the clasp axis *. The path of movement of the indirect retainer is thus directed obliquely, rather than at right angles, to the mucosal surface. This combination of oblique approach and mucosal compression may allow a significant degree of movement of the denture in function.

254 (1) When possible, the indirect retainer should rest on a surface at right angles to the potential path of movement of that indirect retainer. (2) If it rests on an inclined tooth surface, movement of the tooth might occur with resulting loss of support for the indirect retainer.

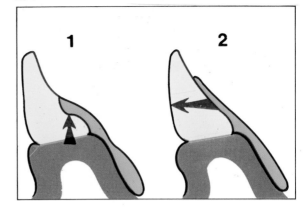

254

Examples of partial denture designs which include indirect retention

Each design is only one of a number of possible solutions.

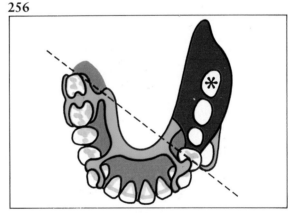

255

255 **Kennedy I.** Indirect retention in this design is provided by incisal rests on 43 and 33.

In this example and in **256** to **258** the part of the saddle susceptible to displacement in an occlusal direction is indicated by an asterisk.

256 **Kennedy II.** Indirect retention in this instance is provided primarily by rests on 44 and 43 as they are furthest from the clasp axis. The rests on 33 and 34 also contribute though to a lesser extent.

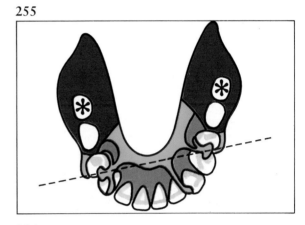

256

257 **Kennedy III.** In the case of bounded saddles there is the potential for direct retention from both abutments. When this can be achieved, as for the saddle replacing 16 and 15, indirect retention is not required. However, it is not uncommon for only one of the abutments to be suitable for clasping. In this design a clasp on 23 has been omitted for aesthetic reasons. Under such circumstances indirect retention can be employed, the major contribution being made by the rest on 17.

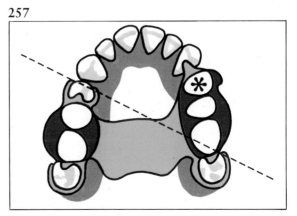

257

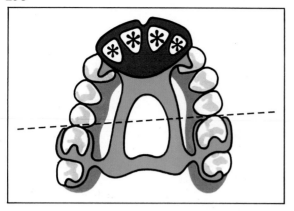

258 Kennedy IV. In an upper denture it is sometimes difficult to achieve much separation of the clasp axis and indirect retainers. In this example, clasps engage the mesiobuccal undercuts on 16 and 26 and indirect retention has been achieved by placing the rests on 17 and 27 as far posteriorly as possible.

An additional function of indirect retainers is to allow accurate location of the partial denture framework against the teeth when undertaking the altered cast procedure (Chapter 25) or when obtaining a wash impression to rebase a free-end saddle.

14 Connectors

259 Connectors are described as being either minor or major. The minor connectors (coloured light blue) join the small components, such as rests and clasps, to the saddles or to the major connector. In addition, they may contribute to the functions of bracing and reciprocation as in the RPI system (**218**). The positioning of the minor connectors joining rests to a saddle will vary according to whether an 'open' or 'closed' design is to be used (**170**). The major connector (coloured black) links the saddles and thus unifies the structure of the denture. The remainder of this chapter is devoted to the major connector.

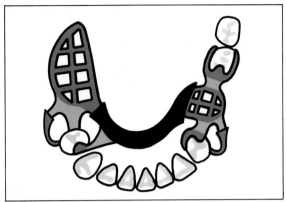

The major connector is capable of fulfilling a number of functions. In addition to its basic connecting role it may play an influential part in retaining the denture by means of extensive mucosal coverage or by engaging guide surfaces, and in providing indirect retention. It certainly is a significant distributor of functional loads in both vertical and horizontal planes and it is in this particular context that we must consider briefly the arguments for and against rigid and non-rigid (stress breaking) connectors.

260 During loading, a component resting on a tooth will be displaced very much less than one which rests on mucosa. If a denture is entirely tooth-supported, the displacement differential between teeth and mucosa is immaterial. The connector should be designed so that it is rigid and thus distributes the functional forces throughout the structure of the denture and thence to the supporting tissues.

260

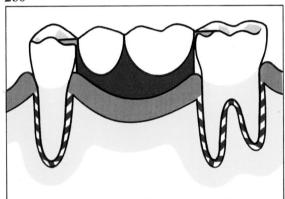

261 A free-end saddle gains some of its support from teeth and some from the tissues of the edentulous area. This support differential will result in tipping of the denture when it is loaded during function, causing an uneven distribution of load over the saddle area. It will also result in a relatively greater share of the load being taken by the tooth. One way of minimising the problem is to compress the denture-bearing mucosa when the impression is taken by using the altered cast impression technique (Chapter 25). In this way some of the displacement distance is taken up and a simple rigid connector can be used in the normal way.

261

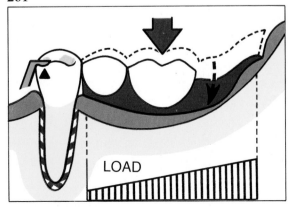

LOAD

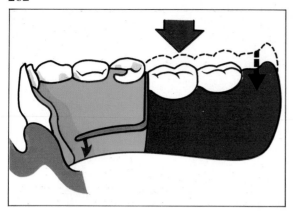

262 An alternative approach is to create a design with 'independent rear suspension' by using a flexible connector such as this split lingual plate. If the saddle component is able to move more than the tooth-supported component, more load will be transmitted to the tissues of the edentulous area and the load will be more evenly distributed. This is the principle governing the stress-broken denture which perhaps has its greatest indication for use in the lower jaw and in cases where the periodontal support for the teeth is relatively poor.

It is not the purpose of this Atlas to rehearse in detail the various arguments for and against rigid and stress-broken connectors. Indeed, some of these arguments are probably of more theoretical interest than of practical value. Inevitably, the stress-broken design is a more complex construction and thus more costly; it may also pose greater demands on plaque control and be less well tolerated by the patient. The use of a rigid connector may make it easier to design a simple shape. For these reasons we are more inclined to prescribe the rigid connector and control the load distribution to the various tissues by reducing the artificial occlusal table, seeking maximum coverage of the tissues of the edentulous areas and using more flexible clasp systems.

Whichever method is used, the long-term health of the denture-bearing tissues is dependent upon careful maintenance of the denture.

Designs of connector for the upper jaw

It is possible to design many shapes of connector. The choice is greater in the upper jaw because of the area available for coverage offered by the palate. It is not our objective to provide a comprehensive catalogue of connectors but rather to present a set of basic principles which act as a guide to the eventual choice of shape.

A decision on design is based upon:
1. functional requirements
2. anatomical constraints
3. ability to fulfil the important criteria of rigidity, hygiene and patient acceptability

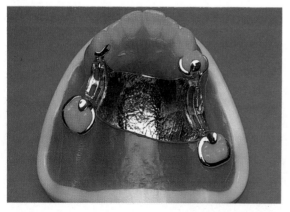

263 An inescapable *functional requirement* is linking the various saddles. Here a simple mid-palatal plate has been used. This connector can easily be made rigid and reduces gingival margin coverage to a minimum. The shape is well tolerated because it can be kept away from the sensitive area around the rugae and incisive papilla. Most of the support and bracing are provided by the abutment teeth and some by the palatal vault.

264 In contrast, the size and distribution of the saddles in this example pose more of a problem. The functional forces can be shared between teeth and palate by utilising a larger connector which extends anteriorly over part of the rugae area and posteriorly to the junction of hard and soft palates. It is still possible to leave the gingival margins of the majority of teeth uncovered.

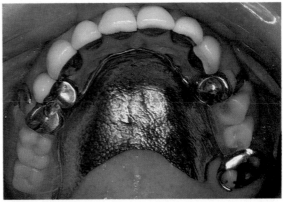

265 Full palatal coverage with cobalt chromium has two disadvantages. First, the bulk of material increases the weight of the appliance. Second, the position of the post-dam cannot be altered should it prove to be poorly tolerated by the patient. An alternative approach is to construct a casting as illustrated. The posterior part is a retaining mesh to which the acrylic denture base will be attached.

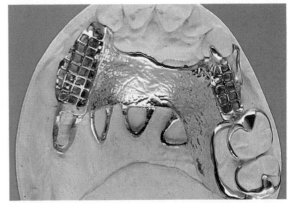

266 If the abutment teeth are healthy and are capable of accepting most of the functional load it is possible to use a 'ring' connector. Less palate is covered but the bars must obviously be thicker than a plate if the connector is to be rigid.

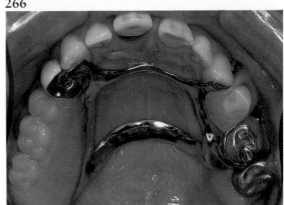

267 Rigidity may be helped if the anterior and posterior bars lie in different planes, thus contributing to an L-shaped girder effect. Whereas some patients appreciate the reduction in coverage, others may have difficulty in tolerating the bulk of metal and the extra length of exposed border of the connector.

The upper jaw poses few *anatomical constraints*, with the exception of a pronounced palatine torus where a 'ring' connector may be the ideal answer.

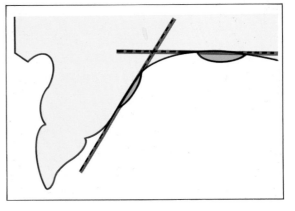

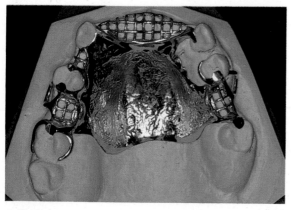

268 Where two or more teeth separate adjacent saddles (23 and 24) it is possible to keep the border of the connector away from the vulnerable gingival margins. Where only one tooth is present (13 or 15) it is often impracticable to uncover the gingival margin. The small slot so created is likely to be tolerated badly by the patient.

269

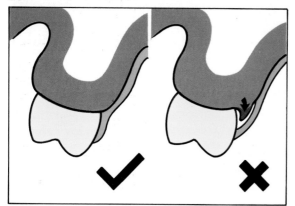

269 If the gingival margin is to be covered totally by the connector, close contact should be achieved whenever possible. If 'gingival relief' is created, the space is soon obliterated by proliferation of the gingival tissue; this change in shape only serves to increase the depth of the periodontal pocket and thus make plaque control that much more difficult.

Designs of connector for the lower jaw

The restricted area for coverage in the lower jaw places a different set of constraints on connector design. In terms of *functional requirements* the connector is more often called upon to distribute some of the load to the natural teeth and may well play an important role in providing indirect retention. The main *anatomical constraint* is the distance between the lingual gingival margin and the functional depth of the floor of the mouth. With gingival recession there is less room to manoeuvre and it may be more difficult to design a connector which satisfies two of the criteria – maintenance of oral hygiene and rigidity.

270

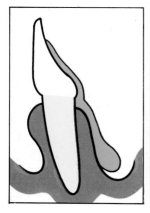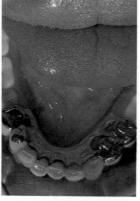

Five of the common connectors are illustrated diagramatically and clinically.

270 The lingual plate covers most of the lingual aspects of the teeth, the gingival margins and the lingual aspect of the ridge. The plate terminates at the functional depth of the sulcus. Rigidity is achieved by thickening the lower border to a bar-like section. One of the major drawbacks of the plate, encouraging plaque formation, has been mentioned previously (**16**).

271 The functional depth of the lingual sulcus is also the inferior limit of the lingual bar. The cross-section of the bar is determined by the shape of the wax pattern either prescribed by the dentist or selected by the dental technician. A lingual bar constructed in cobalt chromium alloy may not be a rigid connector.

272 The combination of lingual bar and continuous clasp (also called a Kennedy bar) is, in essence, the same as a lingual plate with a window cut through it in the region of the gingival margin. Some patients find the two bars irritating to the tongue.

273 The cross-section of the lingual bar is determined empirically. An alternative is to use a sublingual bar whose dimensions are determined by the master impression which records the functional width and depth of the lingual sulcus. In essence, an accurate impression is taken of the sulcus (**399** and **400**) and the available space is filled with the connector. Bearing in mind that the rigidity of a lingual bar increases by a square factor when its height is increased and by a cube factor when its width is increased, it will be appreciated that the increased width of the sublingual bar connector ensures that the important requirement of rigidity is satisfied.

274 On occasions, there is insufficient room between gingival margin and floor of the mouth for either a sublingual or lingual bar. Unless the periodontal health is well maintained, a lingual plate covering the gingival margins might well tip the delicate balance between health and disease. An alternative, where the clinical crowns are long enough, is the dental bar, which is a very substantial continuous clasp. Patient tolerance inevitably places some restriction on its cross-section and thus some reduction in rigidity may have to be accepted.

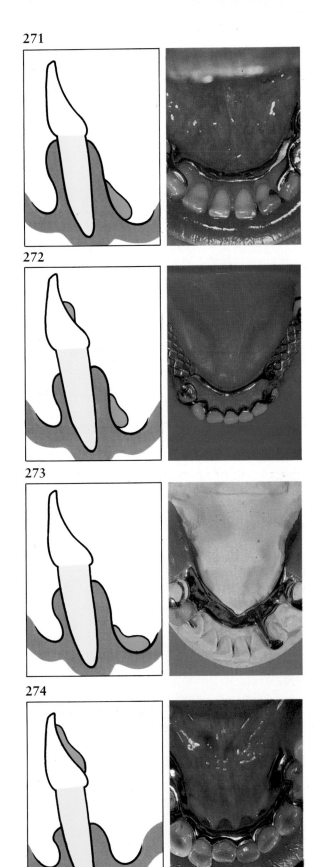

A summary of the functions and essential qualities of the common lower connectors is presented in the accompanying table.

Connector	Connect	Brace	Indirect Retention	Rigidity	Hygiene	Tolerance
Sublingual bar	*			* *	*	*
Lingual bar	*			?	*	*
Lingual bar + continuous clasp	*	*	*	*	*	?
Lingual plate	*	*	*	*	?	*
Dental bar	*	*	*	?	*	?

275

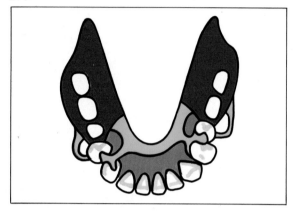

275 If either sublingual or lingual bars are to be used and additional bracing and indirect retention are required, bracing arms and occlusal rests must be added to the design.

Tolerance of the patient must be assessed carefully before prescribing a dental bar or a lingual bar and continuous clasp. Plaque control should be of a high standard before a lingual plate can be prescribed with confidence.

There are more *anatomical constraints* in the lower jaw. Mention has already been made of lack of space between the gingival margin and the floor of the mouth. A prominent lingual fraenum may compound the problem and make it impossible to use a sublingual bar. A mandibular torus (**42**) may be such a size that a sublingual or lingual bar, sitting on top of the bony protuberance, would occupy space in the floor of the mouth to an unacceptable degree.

276

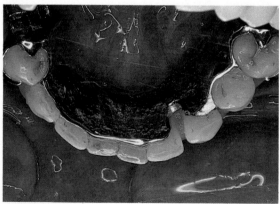

276 Diastemas between the incisors will preclude the use of the dental bar or continuous clasp on aesthetic grounds. Probably the best approach is to prescribe a sublingual bar although a notched lingual plate is an alternative solution.

277 Mention has already been made of lingually inclined teeth (**152**) and how a change in path of insertion can eliminate the obstruction. However, on rare occasions the lingual tilt is so severe that a labial (or buccal) bar has to be used. It will be immediately obvious that a very accurate impression must be taken of the functional depth of the labial sulcus so that the connector can be positioned correctly. The cross-section of the bar will be determined by the space available and also by the patient's tolerance.

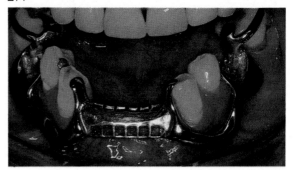

The combination of limited space for the bar and its increased length as it travels around the outer circumference of the dental arch makes it difficult to achieve rigidity although, in this instance, the short spans minimise this problem.

Acrylic dentures

Although most of this Atlas is concerned with the design and construction of dentures with cast metal frameworks, there are occasions when it is appropriate to provide dentures made entirely in acrylic resin.

The major advantages of acrylic resin dentures are their relatively low cost and the ease with which they can be modified. They are therefore most commonly indicated where the life of the denture is expected to be short or where alterations such as additions or relines will be needed; for both these reasons the expense of a metal denture may well be difficult to justify.

Indications for such treatment include:

1 When a denture is required during the phase of rapid bone resorption following tooth loss, for example an immediate denture replacing anterior teeth. In this case a reline followed by early replacement of the denture is to be expected.

2 When a denture must be provided for a young patient where growth of the jaws and development of the dentition are still proceeding.

3 When the remaining teeth have a poor prognosis and their extraction and subsequent addition to the denture is anticipated. A transitional denture may be fitted under such circumstances so that the few remaining teeth can stabilise the prosthesis for a limited period while the patient develops the neuromuscular skills necessary to control the planned replacement complete denture successfully.

4 When a diagnostic (or interim) denture is required before a definitive treatment plan can be formulated. Such an appliance may be required to determine whether an increase in occlusal vertical dimension, required to allow effective restoration of the dentition, can be tolerated by the patient.

In addition, acrylic dentures may also provide a more permanent solution; for example, where only a few isolated teeth remain, an acrylic connector may function at least as well as one in metal.

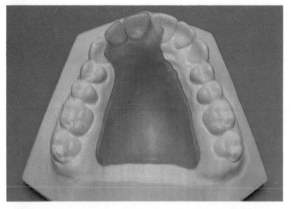

278 Where an acrylic denture is provided as a long-term prosthesis it is particularly important that its potential for tissue damage is minimised by careful design. This is easier to achieve in the upper jaw, where the palate allows extensive mucosal coverage for support and retention without the denture necessarily having to cover the gingival margins. A popular form of design for the replacement of one or two anterior teeth in young people is the 'spoon' denture. It reduces gingival margin coverage to a minimum but a potential hazard is the risk of inhalation or ingestion.

279

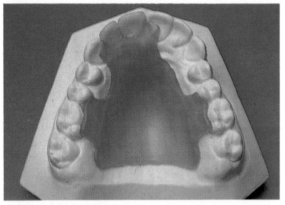

279 A more stable and therefore more acceptable design is the modified spoon denture. Here one has the choice of relying on frictional contact between the connector and the palatal surfaces of some of the posterior teeth or of adding wrought wire clasps.

280

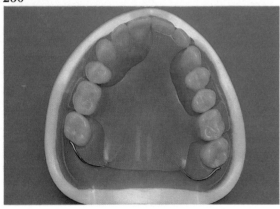

280 Another acceptable design is the 'Every' denture which can be used for restoring multiple bounded saddle areas in the upper jaw. Its characteristics are as follows:
1 All denture borders are at least 3 mm from the gingival margins.
2 The 'open' design of saddle/tooth junction is employed.
3 Point contact between the artificial teeth and abutment teeth is established to reduce lateral stress to a minimum.
4 Posterior wire 'stops' are included to prevent distal drift of the posterior teeth with consequent loss of the contact points.
5 Flanges are included to assist the bracing of the denture.
6 Lateral stresses are reduced by achieving as much balanced occlusion and articulation as possible.

When considering whether or not to provide a partial denture in acrylic resin, the limitations of the material should be borne in mind. This material is weaker and less rigid than the metal alloys and therefore the denture is more likely to flex or fracture during function. To minimise these problems the acrylic connector has to be relatively bulky. This, in turn, can cause problems with tolerance and offers less scope for a design which allows the gingival margins to be left uncovered.

Another significant disadvantage of acrylic resin is that it is radiolucent; location of the prosthesis can prove difficult if the denture is swallowed or inhaled.

15 System of design

It will already be appreciated that a partial denture is the sum of a number of components. In this final chapter of Part 2 we describe a method of building these components into a design and emphasise the importance of prescribing the design to the dental technician.

It must of course be remembered that the design sequence is but one stage of the overall treatment plan for a partially edentulous patient and is undertaken after completing the all-important stages of surveying the cast and selecting a path of insertion.

The following two examples illustrate how to apply the basic principles of design using the following sequence:

1 Saddles
2 Support
3 Retention
4 Bracing and reciprocation
5 Connector
6 Indirect retention

(For easy identification, the various components are illustrated in different colours.)

Example 1

Saddles (yellow)

281 This upper arch has two bounded edentulous areas on the right side and a free-end edentulous area on the left. The teeth have small crowns. 24 is rotated distally. There is no requirement for a labial flange at 13. It has been decided to use a 'closed' design for all three saddles as the short clinical crowns offer limited prospects for clasp retention. The saddle must be fully extended in the free-end edentulous area. Spaced meshwork will be requested for the two posterior saddles to enable them to be relined when required.

Support (red)

282 Tooth support is to be gained on 17, 14 and 24. Because 24 is rotated, a mesial rest would create a major problem of appearance. The occlusal rest is therefore placed on the distal aspect of the tooth. Rest seat preparation is planned for the three teeth. It is apparent that additional support must be gained by palatal coverage.

281

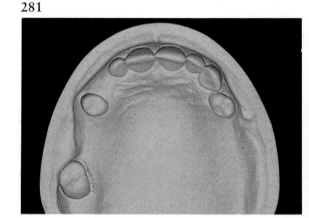

282

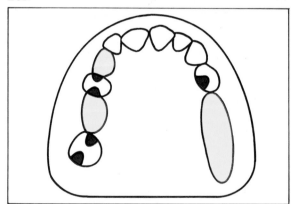

Retention (green)

283 It is practicable and convenient to seek clasp retention on only three teeth (17, 14 and 24). Thus the physical forces of retention must be harnessed by adequate palatal coverage, full extension of the denture base into the left buccal sulcus and around the left tuberosity, and by contact with the guide surfaces which will be prepared on these teeth.

As most of the undercut on 17 is situated on its mesiobuccal aspect, a 'ring' clasp is a suitable design. It is not possible to use a gingivally approaching clasp on 14 because of a bony undercut in the buccal sulcus. As an occlusally approaching clasp is the only reasonable alternative, a wrought gold wire has been chosen as the material that will possess sufficient flexibility for the short arm. As a prominent fraenum precludes a gingivally approaching clasp on 24, a wrought gold occlusally approaching clasp is to be used here also.

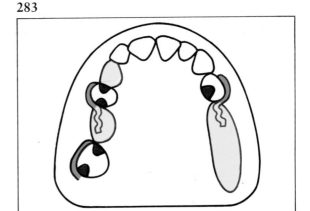

Bracing and reciprocation (blue)

284 It has been decided to obtain bracing from the rigid palatal arm of the 'ring' clasp on 17, by contacting the palatal aspects of 14 and 24 with the connector and by full extension of the free-end saddle. In this instance the bracing components on the teeth will also provide reciprocation to the retentive arms. Retention will also be assisted by the buccal placement of all retentive arms, thus providing cross-arch reciprocation.

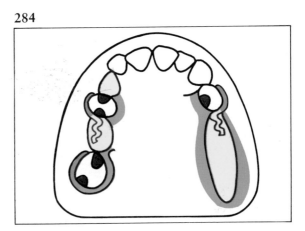

Connector (black)

285 For the reasons given already, widespread palatal coverage is needed. However, it is possible to keep the anterior border of the palatal plate away from the anterior teeth and from the sensitive area around the incisive papilla to promote hygiene and tolerance to the framework.

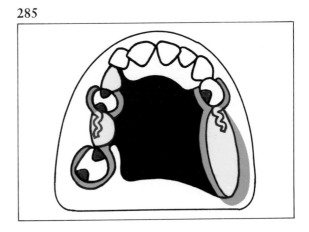

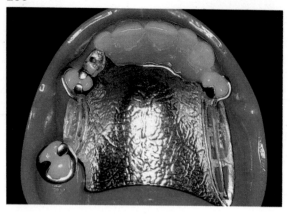

Indirect retention

286 It is necessary to plan for indirect retention to prevent the free-end saddle from moving occlusally. The major clasp axis is sited through 17 and 24. The displacing force will be resisted by the mesial occlusal rest on 14 and by the palatal connector at the front of the mouth.

Design prescription

As the design is being developed at the treatment planning stage, it should be drawn on a proforma to provide easy reference during the preparatory treatment. Once this treatment has been completed, and after the final impression has been obtained, the prescription must be given to the dental technician.

287a

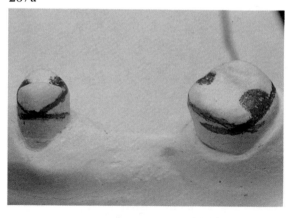

287b

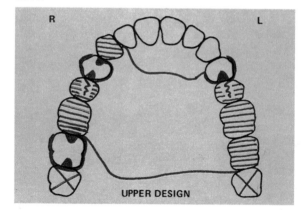

287a and **287b** The design may be drawn on the surveyed master cast using a different coloured lead to that used in the surveyor (**a**). Alternatively (**b**) it can be sent to the laboratory on a proforma although it must be remembered that the shape and extent of the connector can only be prescribed accurately by drawing the outline on the cast.

The prescription must include details of the materials to be used. In this case the dental technician will be asked to construct a cobalt chromium casting with the retentive clasps on 14 and 24 being made from 0.8 mm wrought gold wire.

Example 2

Saddles (yellow)

288 This lower arch has a unilateral free-end edentulous area. A gap exists between 46 and the mesially tilted 48. One lower incisor is missing. A spaced retaining meshwork will be required to enable the saddle to be relined following alveolar resorption. A narrow occlusal table will be used to reduce the load falling on the tissues of the edentulous area. A closed design will be used to provide reciprocation on the distal surface of 34.

Support (red)

289 Tooth support for the saddle will be gained from a mesial occlusal rest on 34. The greatest possible mucosa support for the saddle is achieved by extending the denture base on to the retromolar pad and to the full functional depth of the lingual and buccal sulci. On the right side of the arch it is important to spread the support so that a stable appliance can be produced. The rests have been placed on 44, 46 and 48. The occlusal rests on the molars bridge the gap between the two teeth. Rest seat preparations will be carried out.

Retention (green)

290 The free-end saddle will be carefully shaped to enable the oral musculature to act against the polished surface of the denture. Suitable undercut and sulcus shape allow a gingivally approaching clasp to be used on 34. This clasp will be one of the components for the RPI system and the tooth will be prepared accordingly. On 46 the usable undercut is on the mesiolingual aspect of the tooth and will be engaged by an occlusally approaching clasp.

Bracing and reciprocation (blue)

291 Lateral forces will be transmitted through the minor connectors, through the buccal bracing arm on 46 and to the tissues of the edentulous area through the fully extended flanges. Guide surfaces will be prepared on 34 and 46 to provide reciprocation for the retentive clasps.

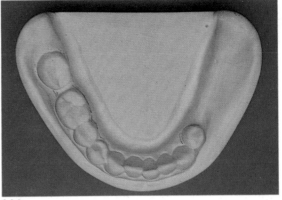

289

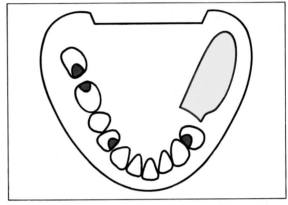

290

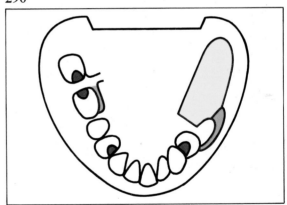

291

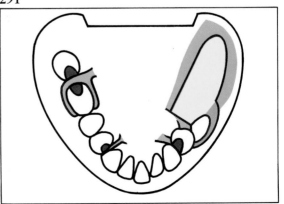

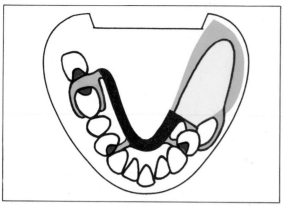

Connector (black)

292 There is sufficient room in the lingual sulcus for a sublingual bar. This connector will be rigid and will reduce coverage of the gingival margins to a minimum. The three minor connectors are placed as unobtrusively as possible in the embrasures between the teeth to ensure that the framework is well tolerated by the patient.

293

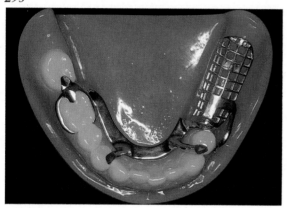

Indirect retention

293 The occlusal rest on 44 will prevent displacement of the free-end saddle in an occlusal direction because it is well positioned in front of the clasp axis passing through 34 and 46. The occlusal rest on 34 will play a minor role in this respect.

294a

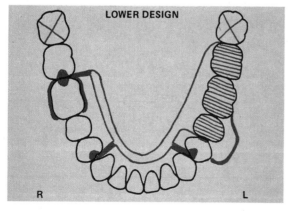

LOWER DESIGN

R   L

294b

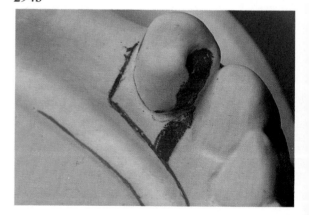

Design prescription

294a and **294b** The same amount of information must be supplied as for Example 1. In this instance the whole casting will be constructed in cobalt chromium alloy. The shape of the sublingual bar is dictated by the shape of the sulcus, which should have been faithfully recorded on the cast. Nevertheless, it is wise to draw the outline of the connector on the cast.

Part 3
Preparation of the mouth

The chapters in Part 3 describe procedures for creating the best possible oral environment for the provision of a partial denture and are arranged in the sequence most commonly appropriate to clinical practice. However, it should be remembered that there will be occasions when several of the procedures are undertaken concurrently or when it is necessary to alter the sequence.

An example of a typical course of treatment might be as follows:–

Impressions for study casts are obtained and a provisional design produced at the outset, because the design of the proposed appliance may well influence, or be influenced by, subsequent treatment such as extractions, orthodontics and the design of tooth restorations. Any treatment required to stabilise the patient's oral condition will also need to be undertaken at the earliest opportunity.

The following items of treatment, if required, should be carried out at an early stage for the reasons indicated:–

1   Initial prosthetic treatment – to overcome the patient's current denture problems.

2   Surgery – to allow the longest possible healing period before new dentures are provided.

3   Periodontal treatment – so that the patient's ability to maintain a high standard of plaque control can be monitored for an adequate period before final decisions are taken concerning the type of denture, if any, to provide. Also, changes in gingival contour following periodontal treatment should be complete before working impressions are obtained.

4   Orthodontic treatment – so that any required improvement in the position of the teeth can be achieved without delaying the prosthetic treatment unduly.

Once the preparatory treatment outlined above has been completed the following items may be required:–

5   Conservation treatment and root canal therapy – to ensure that the remaining teeth are in a good state of repair and that their contours are unlikely to be altered once a partial denture has been constructed.

6   Tooth preparation – so that the crown shape of the remaining teeth is improved to receive rests, retentive clasp arms, bracing and reciprocating elements.

These two aspects of preparatory treatment are closely linked as conservation treatment may be required to achieve the desired crown shape.

16 Initial prosthetic treatment

Initial prosthetic treatment may involve modification of an existing denture or provision of an interim prosthesis as a preparation for the definitive course of treatment.

When modifying existing dentures the following points should be borne in mind. First, as these dentures are commonly due for early replacement, modifications will not have to last for very long. Second, the patient will often be reluctant to part with the denture for the modifications to be carried out, particularly if it replaces anterior teeth. These considerations point to modification of the denture at the chairside wherever practicable. The recent development of a range of polymers for direct use in the mouth has significantly increased the number of opportunities for adopting this approach. Their relatively short clinical life, usually measured in months rather than years, is not a problem where early replacement of the denture is anticipated.

Repairs and additions

Before undertaking a repair it is essential to determine the cause of the fracture so that appropriate corrective measures can be undertaken.

Clasps and rests

295 To replace fractured clasps and rests, or to add these components to a denture, an alginate impression in a stock tray is required of the denture *in situ*. Great care must be taken to ensure that the impression material does not displace the denture from its correct relationship to the surrounding tissues.

Where a component is to be added and the occlusion will influence the design or position of that component, an impression of the opposing dentition is also needed. If it will not be possible to place the casts by hand into the intercuspal position an interocclusal record will be required.

296 A new clasp arm is usually produced by adapting a wrought stainless steel wire to the tooth on the cast and then attaching the wire to the existing acrylic base (1). Alternatively, an entirely new clasp assembly can be cast and tagged into the saddle of the denture (2). This latter procedure would normally be undertaken only if the existing denture is to be used for a considerable time.

295

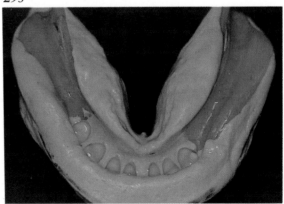

296

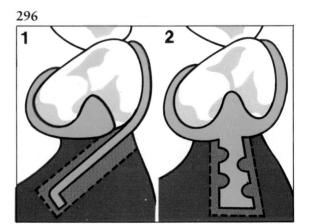

297

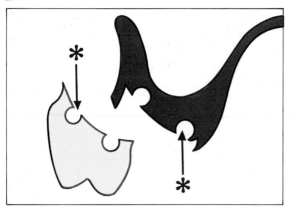

Teeth

297 If a tooth has become detached from the denture but is still available, a rapid chairside repair can usually be effected using cold-curing acrylic resin. It is advisable to cut some form of mechanical retention * in order to reinforce the chemical bond.

The addition of a new artificial tooth may be required to fill a space created either by loss of a denture tooth or by extraction of a natural tooth. This is best done by obtaining an alginate impression and interocclusal records, as described in **295**, so that the addition can be made in the laboratory.

298a

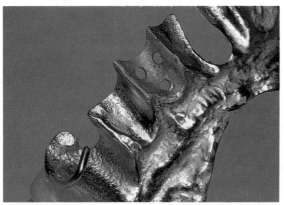

298b

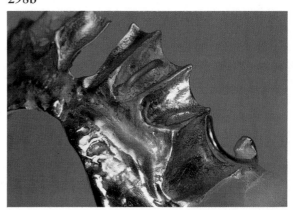

298a and **298b** The attachment of teeth to metal connectors requires the creation of mechanical

retention such as perforations or soldered wire loops.

299

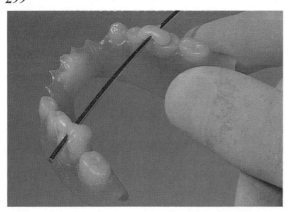

Connectors

299 If the portions of a fractured acrylic denture can be relocated accurately outside the mouth, the clinician can unite them with a wire rod held on to the occlusal surfaces with sticky wax or by applying a cyano-acrylate adhesive to the fracture surfaces. If possible the assembled denture should then be tried in the mouth for accuracy before being sent to the laboratory for repair.

Alternatively, a chairside repair using cold-curing acrylic resin is sometimes possible.

300 If the portions of the denture do not relocate accurately outside the mouth they should be held in the best possible relationship by an application across the fracture line of butyl methacrylate resin or impression compound. The denture may then be seated in the mouth while the bonding material is still pliable, and both portions held in their correct relation to the ridges and teeth until the denture is rigidly united. A laboratory repair can then be undertaken.

If apposition cannot be achieved or if a metal connector is broken or bent the denture will usually have to be remade.

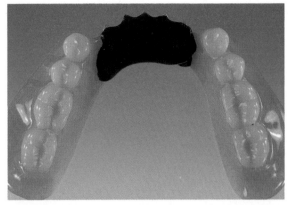

Flanges

301 The addition or extension of a flange may be achieved using a butyl methacrylate resin which is adaptable directly in the mouth. However, as the colour stability of these resins is relatively poor, the technique is not ideal if the flange is visible and the denture is to be worn for more than a few weeks.

For the laboratory addition of a flange, an alginate impression is taken of the denture *in situ* with a stock tray which has been carefully border moulded with compound in the area where the flange is to be added.

301

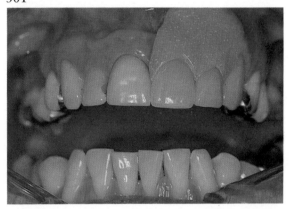

302 Alternatively, a border moulding material such as tracing compound can be added to the denture and shaped to conform to the area to be covered by the flange. A local wash impression is then taken within the modified flange.

302

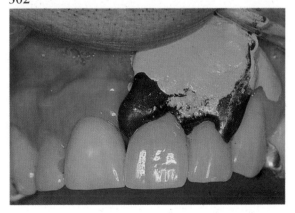

Temporary relining

A denture may be relined temporarily where loss of fit has resulted in instability or mucosal injury.

Temporary relining is carried out in the mouth using either soft or hard materials. When mucosal inflammation is present the cushioning effect of the soft materials (tissue conditioners) is an advantage in that it distributes the load more evenly and thus promotes healing. The hard materials are cold-curing acrylic resins with either butyl or methyl methacrylate monomer. The former has the advantage of being less irritating to the oral mucosa.

Before undertaking a temporary reline preparatory adjustment of the denture is commonly necessary.

303

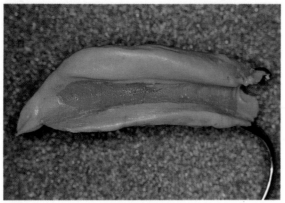

303 A diagnostic alginate impression taken in the old denture is a quick and useful aid to assessing the fit of the denture and identifies pressure points which require adjustment before adding the reline material.

304

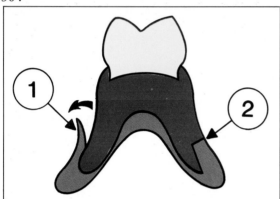

304 If the denture is to be relined any areas of underextension should first be corrected by border moulding with a high viscosity butyl methacrylate resin. This resin does not have a very strong bond to the acrylic denture base and if allowed to form a feather edge (1) at the junction between the two materials will tend to lift and consequently traumatise the oral mucosa. This is prevented if a butt joint (2) is produced between the two resins.

305

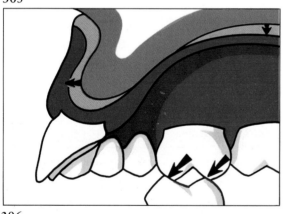

305 When carrying out a direct reline with a temporary material it is all too easy to fail to seat the denture correctly. This is particularly so in the case of an upper denture. If this occurs both the vertical and the horizontal occlusal relationships will be altered. It will also result in thickening of the connector leading to possible problems of patient tolerance and may alter the position of an anterior saddle to an unacceptable degree. These changes are likely to make the denture unwearable.

306

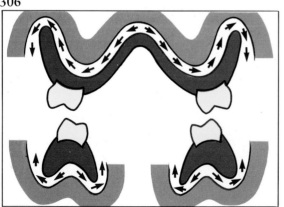

306 There are a number of precautions that can be taken to reduce the chance of the denture being seated incorrectly.

In an upper denture with extensive palatal coverage the escape channel for any excess reline material is long and tortuous and therefore the choice of a low viscosity material is important. In the lower jaw, and in individual saddles, the escape channel is much shorter and so a higher viscosity material may be used.

307 Alternatively, when a lining material of relatively high viscosity such as butyl methacrylate resin is required, escape of the lining material from an upper denture can be helped by drilling holes into the palatal connector and the flanges.

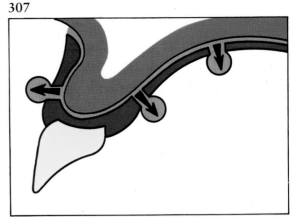

308 Where the loss of fit is localised to the site of recent extractions the temporary reline can be restricted to that area. The remaining, unmodified impression surface helps to locate the denture correctly against the residual ridges and abutment teeth. There will be a line of demarcation between the new resin and the original impression surface but minor smoothing of this junction is all that is usually required to achieve an acceptable result.

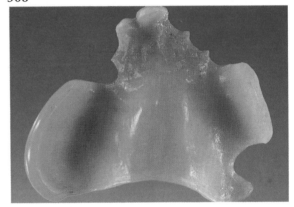

309 If a rigid reline material is being used it is important to appreciate that it may flow into undercut areas around the teeth and that consequently the timing of removal of the denture from the mouth is critical. Failure to remove the denture before curing is complete will result in the denture being locked into place. Removal of the denture will then only be possible if the offending acrylic resin is cut away with burs, a thoroughly time-consuming and frustrating business.

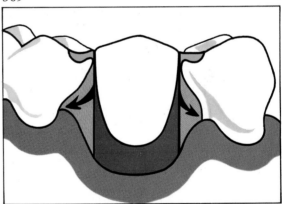

310 Once the denture has been relined, any excess material must be removed from the polished surfaces and teeth. If the relining material is a hard resin the borders are trimmed and polished (upper denture).

Excess tissue conditioner is trimmed on the polished surface of the denture so that the denture border consists of a smooth roll of the conditioning material (lower denture).

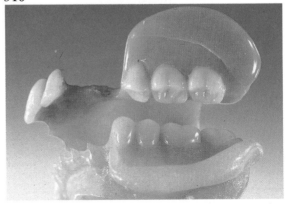

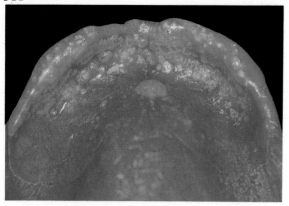

311 A patient who has had a denture relined with a tissue conditioner should be given specific instructions on how to clean the lining. Certain tissue conditioners are damaged by the alkaline perborate denture cleansers and others by the alkaline hypochlorites. Unless the patient is warned of these incompatibilities rapid deterioration of the lining will occur.

As all these linings are added as a temporary measure, a positive decision must be taken by the dentist as to the next stage of treatment. For example, a tissue conditioner needs to be assessed at weekly intervals and replaced periodically until mucosal inflammation has resolved. A new denture can then be constructed.

Occlusal adjustment

312

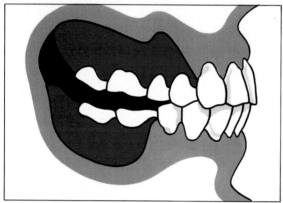

312 The most common occlusal deterioration in dentures which have been worn for many years is loss of occlusal contact resulting from a combination of occlusal wear and sinking of the denture following alveolar resorption. Correction of the occlusion is desirable before constructing replacement dentures as adaptive mandibular posture and mucosal inflammation resulting from this deterioration are likely to interfere with successful treatment.

313

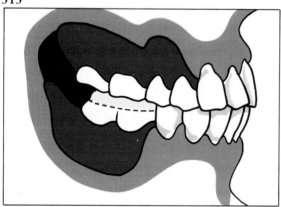

313 After the saddles have been relined, occlusal contact can be re-established by the addition of tooth-coloured cold-curing acrylic resin to the posterior teeth.

The fluid resin is applied to the occlusal surfaces of one of the dentures and allowed to reach the dough stage before the denture is inserted into the mouth. Petroleum jelly is applied to any opposing denture teeth and the mandible is gently guided along the retruded arc of closure until even occlusal contact is made at the appropriate vertical dimension. The denture is then removed from the mouth and the resin allowed to cure before refining the occlusion by selective grinding.

Interim prostheses

An interim prosthesis may be constructed before the definitive denture for the following reasons:

Space maintenance and aesthetics

314

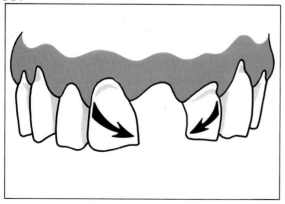

314 The loss of an anterior tooth may require rapid replacement with an interim denture both for social reasons and to prevent reduction of the space by drifting and tilting of the adjacent teeth.

Improving patient tolerance

315 A small minority of patients find it very difficult, or even impossible, to wear a denture because of a pronounced retching reflex. The provision of a thin acrylic training base, which in the upper jaw may be of horseshoe design, is useful in overcoming the reflex. The patient wears the base for increasing periods each day until tolerance is good enough to indicate that conventional treatment can proceed. When a training base of horseshoe design is used, the palatal extension can be increased in stages to allow progressive adaptation to palatal coverage which is as close as possible to the optimum.

In this instance the training base incorporates occlusal coverage in order to modify the jaw relationship in preparation for advanced restorative treatment (see below).

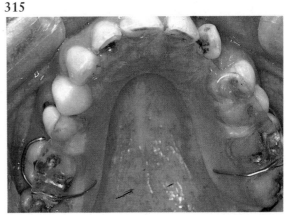

Preparation for advanced restorative treatment

A factor vital to the success of advanced restorative treatment is the ability of the patient to maintain a high level of plaque control. The use of an interim prosthesis will permit a careful evaluation of the oral and denture hygiene over a prolonged period before definitive treatment is commenced.

Advanced prosthetic treatment can fail because of a patient's unrealistic expectation of what a removable prosthesis can achieve, creating dissatisfaction and rejection of the treatment that has been undertaken. The provision of an interim prosthesis gives the patient experience of the limitations of such dentures; this experience, when combined with careful explanation of future treatment aims and expectations, helps to create a more realistic frame of mind and readier acceptance of the definitive prosthesis.

Modifying jaw relationships

Adaptive changes in the jaw relationship may result from loss of teeth, the excessive loss of tooth substance, or the congenital absence of teeth. These changes may require correction before restorative treatment can be undertaken and this may be achieved by the progressive occlusal adjustment of an interim prosthesis until the optimum occlusal relationship is determined.

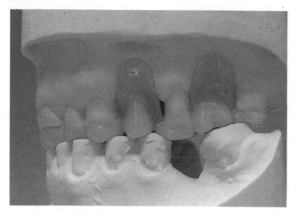

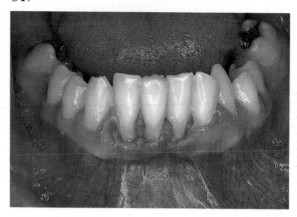

316 The planning of restorations for severely worn teeth is complicated by the uncertainty as to whether the increase in occlusal vertical dimension necessary to accommodate the required restorations will be tolerated by the patient.

An interim prosthesis is constructed to an occlusal height that appears from the initial assessment to be appropriate. It may then be progressively adjusted over several appointments. This allows a period in which the patient can gradually adapt to progressive modest increases in occlusal height and finally confirms a height on which future treatment planning can be based.

317 An interim denture can be helpful in patients exhibiting gingival trauma as a result of a deep incisal overbite.

A simple appliance with a palatal table can provide instant relief while a decision is being taken on the definitive solution whether it be orthodontic, restorative, periodontal or surgical.

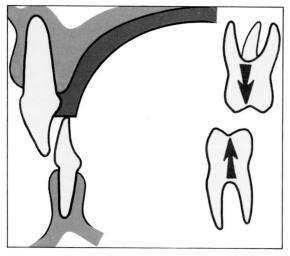

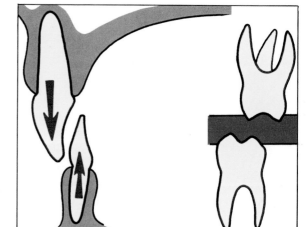

318 In the young patient the palatal table may also improve the situation by allowing further eruption of the posterior teeth and causing some intrusion of the lower anterior teeth.

319 Prevention of gingival trauma should not be achieved with an onlay appliance covering only the posterior teeth as continued eruption of the anterior teeth may result in the original traumatic relationship becoming re-established.

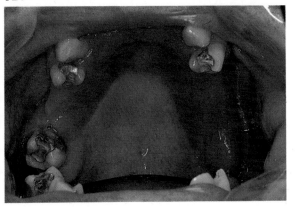

Treatment of denture stomatitis

320 Denture stomatitis is a diffuse inflammation of the denture-bearing mucosa, often of multiple aetiology.

The commonest causes are trauma from the denture and an overgrowth of the fungus *Candida albicans* encouraged by poor denture plaque control. Systemic conditions, such as diabetes, deficiencies of iron, vitamin B12 or folic acid, and drug therapy, including broad-spectrum antibiotics, steroids and cytotoxic agents, may predispose to denture stomatitis.

Treatment of the condition to achieve resolution of the inflammation and the associated mucosal swelling should be carried out before working impressions are obtained.

321

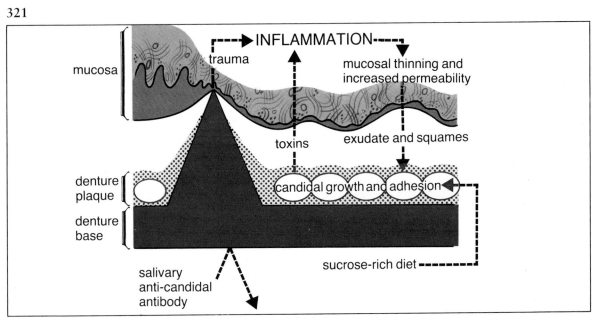

321 Some of the many aetiological and predisposing factors which may play a part in the pathogenesis of denture stomatitis are shown in the figure. The possible interaction of the various factors is complex but a possible scenario is as follows. Trauma from the denture initiates an inflammatory reaction. Thinning of the mucosa results in increased permeability and escape of inflammatory exudate. The exudate, together with desquamated mucosal cells, forms a favourable nutrient medium which promotes the growth of *Candida albicans*. In addition, this exudate, and the sucrose-rich diet which may result from the dietary selection sometimes associated with the wearing of dentures, may contribute to the condition by increasing the adhesiveness of the *Candida* cells, and thus encouraging the formation of denture plaque. As candidal proliferation occurs the rate of production of potent toxins by the micro-organisms increases. The passage of these toxins into the tissues is facilitated by the thinning and increased permeability of the mucosa. Aggravation of the inflammatory response occurs and so a vicious circle is set up. Anti-candidal antibody is secreted in parotid saliva but access of antibody to the *Candida* cells may be restricted by the denture base.

322

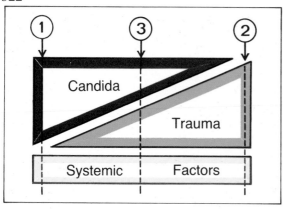

322 The aetiological factors may act alone or in combination as indicated here diagrammatically – in patient (1) the lesion is due to a proliferation of *Candida* organisms, in patient (2) to denture trauma, and in patient (3) to a combination of these factors.

The position of each denture stomatitis patient on this aetiological scale should be estimated so that the appropriate treatment can be carried out.

323

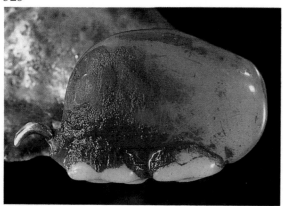

323 If the denture plaque control is poor the dentist should demonstrate the plaque to the patient by the use of a disclosing solution, explain the significance of the plaque and give instruction in how best to remove it.

324

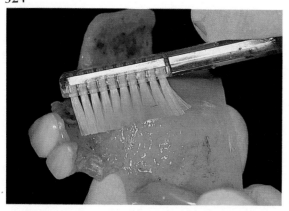

324 To clean the denture the patient should be advised to use a small-headed medium nylon multi-tufted toothbrush which gives good access to all parts of the denture and good adaptability to the surface. Any agent used with the brush should have a low abrasivity for acrylic resin. Soap is one such agent. It should be noted that many proprietary toothpastes and even some denture pastes contain abrasive particles which can damage acrylic resin.

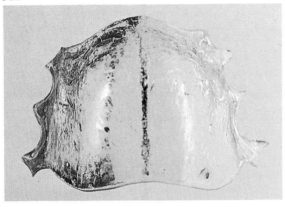

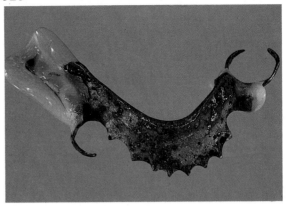

325 Acrylic dentures should also be immersed daily in a cleanser of the hypochlorite type which have been shown to be the most effective chemical agents for plaque removal. An acrylic plate carrying disclosed plaque has been partially immersed for 20 minutes in such a cleanser. The immersed portion (right side) has been rendered plaque-free.

326 Cobalt chromium dentures should not be immersed for long periods in hypochlorite cleansers because there is a risk of corrosion of the metal.

If trauma appears to be a contributory factor to the stomatitis, appropriate adjustments, such as occlusal correction and temporary relining, should be made to the denture as described in the earlier sections of this chapter. It is also advisable under such circumstances for the patient to leave the denture out as much as possible.

If the lesion does not respond to these local measures the investigation of possible systemic factors should be undertaken. In such refractory cases oral antifungal agents such as Amphotericin B, Nystatin or Miconazole may be beneficial. It should be noted, however, that these antifungal agents by themselves are of very limited value and unless the underlying cause of the denture stomatitis is eradicated the condition will recur when the antifungal agents are withdrawn.

17 Surgery

Surgery may be necessary prior to partial denture construction to remove retained roots or unerupted teeth which are superficially located in edentulous areas and to eliminate any pathology associated with teeth or dental remnants. It may also be necessary to improve the contours of edentulous areas by reducing bony prominences and hyperplastic soft tissue and to eliminate prominent fraenal attachments.

327

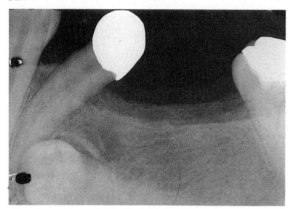

327 This radiograph reveals that an unerupted second premolar has influenced the alignment of the first premolar which is tilted distally and is unsuitable for use as an abutment. If a partial denture is to be provided it will be necessary to consider removal of both teeth.

328

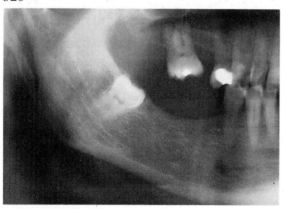

328 A third molar erupting at such an unfavourable angulation will not provide acceptable support for a partial denture and will prevent full extension of the free-end saddle. It should be removed prior to denture construction.

329

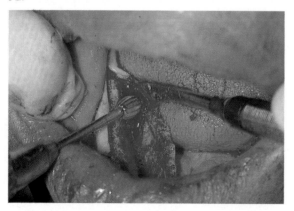

329 Prominent mandibular tori constitute an obstruction to the insertion of a partial denture framework and to the correct location of a lingual connector. Surgical reduction is a relatively simple procedure.

330

330 Bulbous and mobile tuberosities provide poor support for partial denture saddles and may also create problems in the orientation of the occlusal plane. Surgical reduction will improve the contour and consistency of the soft tissues.

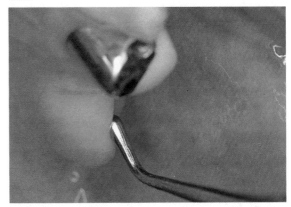

331

331 This localised area of soft tissue hyperplasia has been caused by the prolonged wearing of an unsatisfactory denture. The tissue must be removed before a new denture is constructed. The excised piece of soft tissue should be sent for histopathological examination.

Surgery is clearly indicated in this instance. Where a lesion is associated with the flange of a denture the flange should be cut back to allow resolution of the inflammation before the need for surgery is assessed.

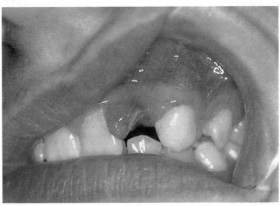

18 Periodontal treatment

Numerous studies have demonstrated that the wearing of partial dentures will tend to encourage the accumulation of plaque. It is important to establish a condition of health in the periodontal tissues prior to prosthetic treatment and to ensure that patients receive detailed instruction in oral hygiene procedures so that the accumulation of plaque around abutment teeth and partial denture components is kept to a minimum.

All patients will therefore require oral hygiene instruction and many will also need basic periodontal treatment. More extensive procedures may also be required on some occasions.

332

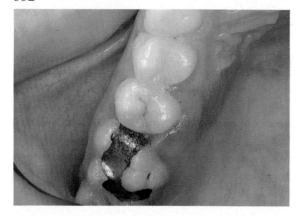

332 Even in a superficially clean mouth the wearing of a partial denture is often associated with some degree of gingival and mucosal inflammation. Localised inflammatory changes of this type will usually resolve if the level of plaque control and denture hygiene can be improved.

333

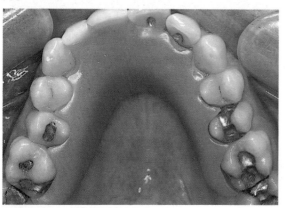

333 This acrylic partial denture which replaces two upper incisors, 12 and 11, has extensive and unnecessary coverage of palatal gingival margins.

334

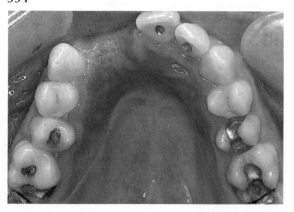

334 Removal of the denture reveals widespread marginal gingivitis and some degree of inflammation of the palatal mucosa. The gingival margins should be exposed, either by modifying the existing denture or by providing an interim prosthesis. Plaque control is then likely to be more effective and the condition should resolve prior to the construction of a well-designed cobalt chromium partial denture.

335 In contrast, there has been so much inflammation and soft tissue damage in this mouth that improvement in oral and denture hygiene is unlikely to achieve resolution. The gingival tissues will need to be recontoured surgically prior to the construction of a replacement partial denture.

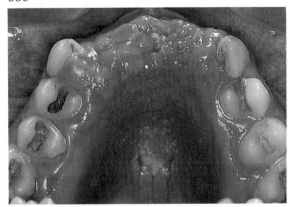

336 Here the inflammatory changes affecting the palatal gingival tissues under a succession of mucosa-borne partial dentures have produced some degree of hypertrophy with pocketing and an unfavourable tissue morphology.

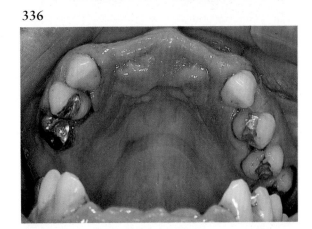

337 A gingivectomy has been undertaken to improve the soft tissue contours, the standard of oral hygiene has been greatly improved and a tooth-supported cobalt chromium partial denture, incorporating generous clearance of the gingival margins, has been provided.

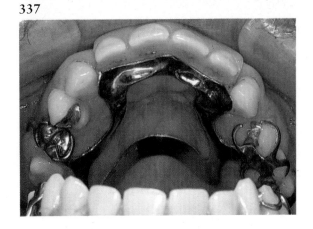

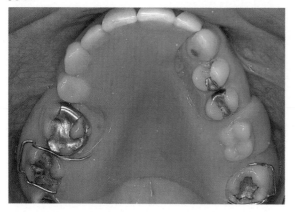

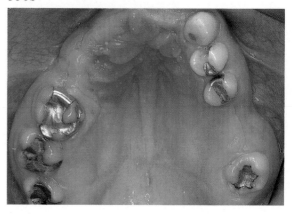

338a The extent and distribution of the edentulous spaces in this mouth makes it difficult to avoid some coverage of gingival margins and this patient has worn a succession of acrylic partial dentures with full palatal coverage. The interim denture shown here has reduced gingival coverage to a minimum.

338b Removal of the denture reveals that the health of the gingival tissue has improved and that there is now only a very mild degree of inflammation affecting the mucosa in the palatal vault.

339

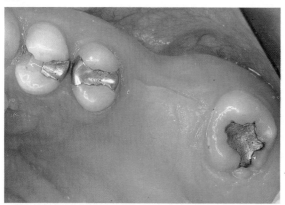

339 Hypertrophy of the gingival tissues, however, has led to coverage of most of the palatal aspect of the crown of 27 and if this tooth is to serve as an abutment for an improved design of partial denture it will be necessary to undertake gingivectomy to expose the anatomical crown. The defective restoration in 24 will of course also require to be replaced.

340

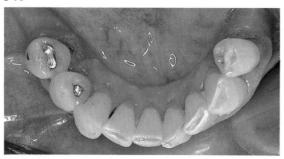

340 This patient has worn a mucosa-borne partial denture in the lower jaw with acrylic free-end saddles and a stainless steel lingual bar connector. This inadequate prosthesis has caused considerable damage to the gingival tissues around 45 and 34, stripping them away from the distal and lingual aspects of these abutment teeth. Deposits of supra- and subgingival calculus are present and 45 shows increased mobility.

It is important to evaluate whether or not the gingival tissues can be restored to a condition of health and whether these teeth now have sufficient investing bone to contribute to the support of a partial denture framework.

19 Orthodontic treatment

Orthodontic treatment has some benefits to offer when partial dentures are required and the space available for the prosthesis has become restricted due to movement of the adjacent teeth. This may happen when some of the permanent teeth fail to develop or erupt or when the presence of an unrestored edentulous gap has allowed some drifting and tilting of the abutments to take place.

341

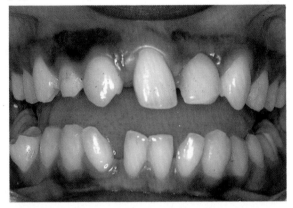

341 In this instance, absence of the permanent maxillary lateral incisors together with early loss of 21 has allowed the remaining central incisor to drift across the midline. Prosthetic treatment has not achieved a satisfactory aesthetic result.

342

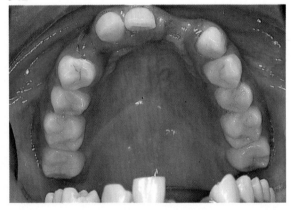

342 The retained deciduous canine has been extracted and a removable orthodontic appliance has been used to retract 11 and bring it into a more acceptable alignment.

343

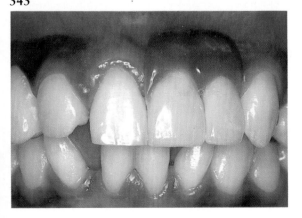

343 The labial and incisal surfaces of 13 and 11 have been recontoured and a partial denture has been provided to produce a more acceptable appearance.
  Further orthodontic treatment is now proposed in order to realign the mandibular dentition.

344

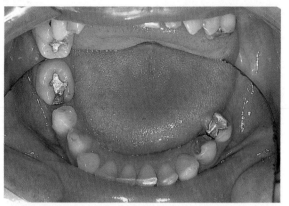

344 Lack of a prosthetic replacement for missing posterior teeth has allowed this lower molar to tilt mesially. In this position it not only offers less than adequate support for a partial denture but creates problems in the maintenance of an adequate standard of oral hygiene.

345

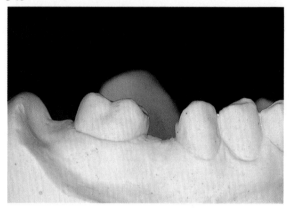

345 Orthodontic treatment has re-established space by uprighting the tooth, and has produced an abutment which offers the possibility of adequate support and retention for a partial denture framework.

There are times when it is necessary to provide permanent retention of teeth following orthodontic treatment and this may involve the use of a partial denture. It is usually more appropriate, however, to use fixed retainers for this purpose.

20 Conservative treatment

Conservative treatment will necessarily precede the construction of dentures in order to ensure that the clinical integrity of the remaining teeth is established before master impressions are recorded. In this way it should be possible to ensure that the accurate fit of the components of the partial denture against the abutment teeth is maintained throughout the life of the denture. There are few procedures more frustrating than to embark on conservative treatment of teeth to which a partial denture framework has already been fitted.

In many cases, requirements of the partial denture design such as support, retention and bracing will necessitate modification of tooth surfaces and the details of such tooth preparations are presented in Chapter 21. Frequently, however, these factors also dictate the form of individual restorations. It is therefore essential that a provisional denture design should be established before details of conservative treatment are finalised.

346

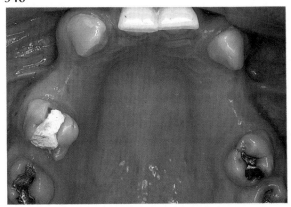

346   It is particularly important that teeth which are to serve as abutments for a partial denture should be carefully evaluated. Here, 16 has advanced caries of the crown structure. It is important to ascertain whether or not it is vital and, if non-vital, to assess whether it has been or can be adequately root treated. It is also critical to ensure that the coronal structure can be soundly restored. If the long-term prognosis is doubtful it may be wiser to consider extraction and incorporation within the partial denture.

347

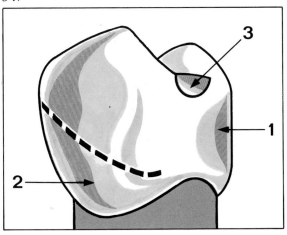

347   Where the need for extensive restoration of a tooth justifies the fitting of a full veneer crown, the opportunity should be taken to incorporate (1) guide surfaces, (2) retentive undercuts and (3) rest seats into the crown. These modifications will usually be carried out at the waxing-up stage of crown construction and will be produced by careful shaping of the wax pattern on the surveyor. However, it must be remembered when preparing the tooth that sufficient tooth structure must be removed to allow these features to be included within the bulk of the restoration.

348

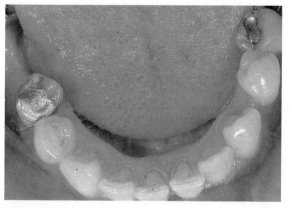

348 The buccal cusp of 45 has recently fractured and the tooth has been restored with a large pinned amalgam restoration. If it is now to serve as a partial denture abutment there is a risk of fracture of the tooth or restoration from the additional load transmitted by the denture components. For this reason it will be restored with a full veneer crown.

349

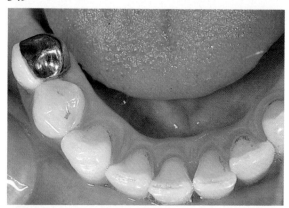

349 The completed restoration incorporates a seat for an occlusal rest that will provide support for a partial denture.

350

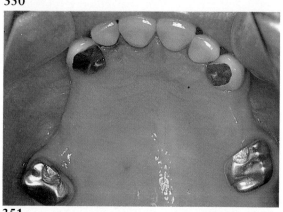

350 Full veneer crowns have been used to reduce the degree of undercut on the buccal aspect of these two upper molars and to provide a more favourable survey line for clasping.

351

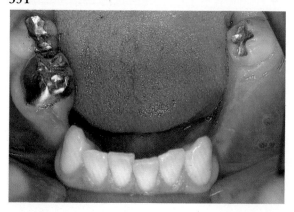

351 In the mandible the need is more frequently to modify lingual contours. Here a crown has been used to reduce an excessive lingual undercut and thus produce a more favourable shape for clasping.

A similar procedure may on occasion be necessary on lingually tilted molars or premolars which would otherwise prevent the insertion of a lingual connector.

352 A lower premolar with an unsatisfactory survey line has been restored with a full veneer crown which provides an acceptable degree of undercut for a gingivally approaching 'I' bar.

Guide surfaces have also been established to determine the path of insertion and removal of the partial denture framework and to provide reciprocation for the retentive clasp arm.

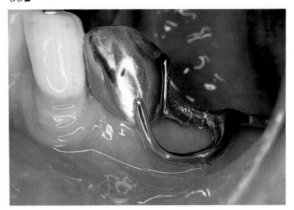

21 Tooth preparation

Preparation may be undertaken for a number of reasons:

1 To provide rest seats.
2 To establish guide surfaces.
3 To modify unfavourable survey lines.
4 To create retentive areas.

In addition, occlusal adjustment may also form an important part of tooth preparation (**81, 82** and **84**).

Tooth preparation for partial dentures should be planned on articulated study casts after they have been surveyed and a denture design produced.

Shaping of enamel surfaces for any of the reasons listed is usually undertaken with rotary diamond instruments of appropriate size and shape. The resulting roughened enamel surface must always be smoothed and polished. Special burs, stones and abrasive-impregnated rubber wheels and points are available for this purpose. Subsequent application of a topical fluoride varnish to reduce the chance of carious attack of the modified enamel surfaces should be carried out routinely.

Rest seats

Rest seats may need to be prepared:

1 to produce a favourable tooth surface for support (**353**),

2 to prevent interference with the occlusion (**354**),
3 to reduce the prominence of a rest (**355**).

353

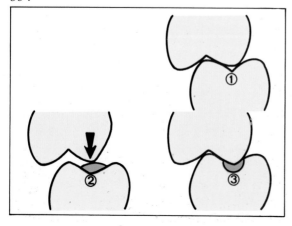

353 A rest placed on an inclined surface will tend to slide down the tooth under the influence of occlusal loads (1). The resulting horizontal force may cause a limited labial migration of the tooth with consequent further loss of support for the denture.

The provision of a rest seat (2) will result in a vertical loading of the tooth, more efficient support and absence of tooth movement.

354

354 An occlusal rest placed at (1) would create a premature occlusal contact (2) unless a rest seat were prepared to make room for it (3).

Space for the rest should not usually be created by grinding the upper palatal cusp as this is a supporting cusp contributing to the stability of the intercuspal position.

355 In addition, a rest placed on an unprepared tooth surface (1) will stand proud of that surface and may thus tend to collect food particles and possibly create difficulties in tolerating the denture.

The preparation of a rest seat (2) will allow the rest to be shaped so that it blends into the contour of the tooth and is less apparent to the patient.

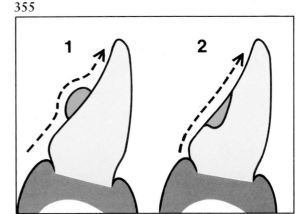

Rest seats on posterior teeth

356 The design of rest seats on posterior teeth is shown in:

1 occlusal view,
2 mesiodistal view,
3 proximal view.

It will be seen that preparation involves a reduction in the height of the marginal ridge in order to ensure an adequate bulk of material linking the occlusal rest to the minor connector.

Rest seats on posterior teeth should normally be saucer-shaped so that a certain amount of horizontal movement of the rest within the seat is possible. Dissipation of some of the energy developed by occlusal forces acting on the denture can then occur.

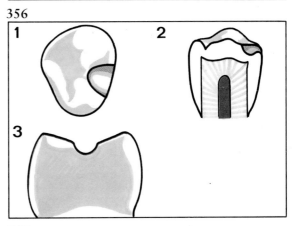

357 The use of a box-shaped rest seat within a cast restoration may result in the rest applying damaging horizontal loads on the abutment tooth. These rest seats should be restricted to tooth-supported dentures where the periodontal health of the abutment teeth is good.

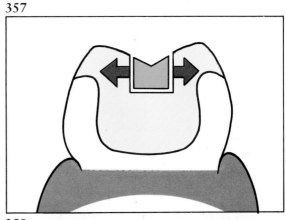

358 The rest should be at least 1 mm thick for adequate strength. To check that sufficient enamel has been removed during rest seat preparation to accommodate this thickness of metal, the patient should be asked to occlude on a strip of softened pink wax. The thickness of wax in the region of the rest seat will indicate if adequate clearance has been achieved.

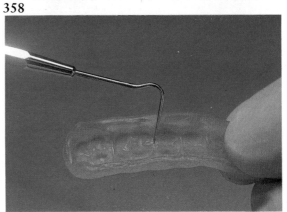

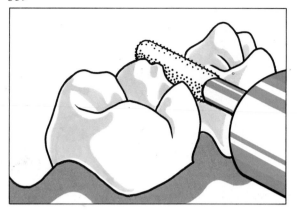

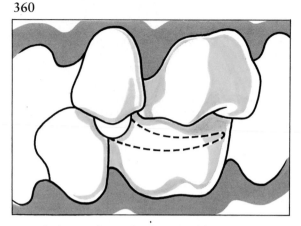

359 and 360 Where a clasp is to extend buccally from an occlusal rest and there is no space occlusally for it to do so, the preparation must be

extended as a channel on to the buccal surface of the tooth.

361

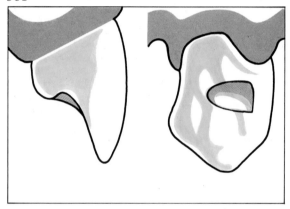

Rest seats on anterior teeth

The design of rest seats on anterior teeth is shown in **361** to **364**.

361 On upper anterior teeth, particularly canines, the cingulum is often well enough developed so that modest preparation to accentuate its form creates a rest seat without penetration of the enamel.

362

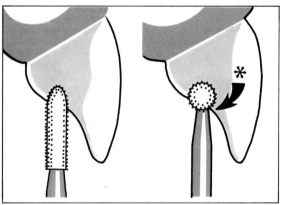

362 A cylindrical diamond stone with a rounded tip should be used to prepare the rest seat. A spherical instrument tends to create unwanted undercuts *.

363 The lingual surface of a lower anterior tooth is usually too vertical and the cingulum too poorly developed to allow preparation of a cingulum rest seat without penetration of the enamel. Incisal rest seats therefore have a wider application in this situation in spite of their inferior appearance. The preparation is shown from the labial (1), lingual (2) and proximal (3) viewpoints.

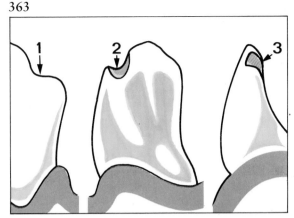

364 Incisal rest seats can be prepared using a tapered cylindrical diamond.

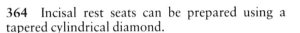

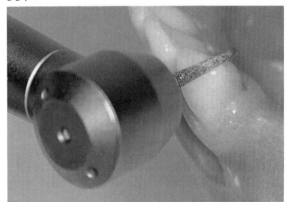

Guide surfaces

365 Guide surfaces * are two or more parallel axial surfaces on abutment teeth which limit the path of insertion of a denture. Guide surfaces may occur naturally or, as is more often the case, may need to be prepared.

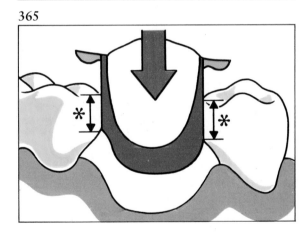

The advantages of guide surfaces

It is widely accepted on the basis of clinical observation that the utilisation of guide surfaces confers a number of benefits in partial denture construction. The benefits include:

1 Increased stability
2 Reciprocation
3 Prevention of clasp deformation
4 Appearance

366

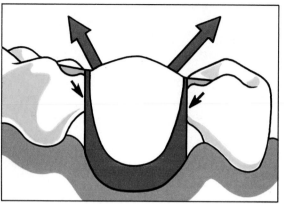

Increased stability

366 This is achieved by the guide surfaces resisting displacement of the denture (red arrows) in directions other than along the planned path of displacement.

367

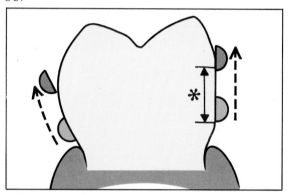

Reciprocation

367 A guide surface * allows a reciprocating component to maintain continuous contact with a tooth as the denture is displaced occlusally. The retentive arm of the clasp is thus forced to flex as it moves up the tooth. It is this elastic deformation of the clasp which creates the retentive force (Chapter 12).

368

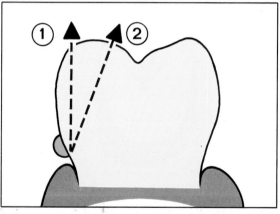

Prevention of clasp deformation

368 Guide surfaces ensure that the patient removes the denture along a planned path (1). The clasps are therefore flexed to the extent for which they were designed.

Without guide surfaces the patient may tilt or rotate the denture on removal (2), causing clasps to flex beyond their proportional limit.

369

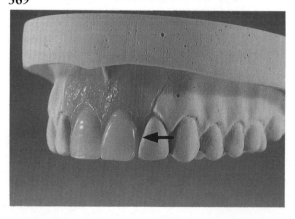

Appearance

369 A guide surface on an anterior abutment tooth permits an intimate contact between saddle and tooth which allows the one to blend with the other, creating a convincing, natural appearance. Guide surfaces often occur naturally in this situation so that tooth preparation is not required.

The preparation of guide surfaces

Guide surfaces are usually prepared somewhat imprecisely by eye. The position in which the handpiece must be held to prepare the required guide surfaces, so that they are all parallel to each other and to the path of insertion, should be established on the study cast.

As a check on the accuracy of the prepared guide surface, an alginate impression may be taken to produce a second study cast. This cast can then be placed on a surveyor and the parallelism of the guide surfaces checked using the analysing rod. If correction is found to be needed, further intra-oral adjustment can be undertaken.

A more precise approach to the preparation of guide surfaces can be achieved by the use of jigs constructed on a prepared study cast and then transferred to the mouth, either to control the positioning of the handpiece or to check on the location and amount of enamel reduction.

370 A guide surface should extend vertically for about 3 mm and should be kept as far from the gingival margin as possible.

370

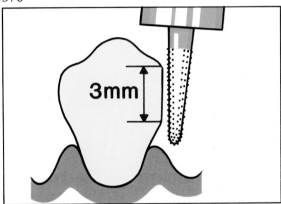

371

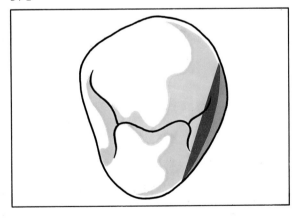

371 A guide surface should be produced by removing a minimal and fairly uniform thickness of enamel, usually not more than 0.5 mm, from around the appropriate part of the circumference of the tooth (green area).

The surfaces should not be prepared as a flat plane as would tend to occur if an abrasive disc were used (red area). This is unnecessarily destructive and may even lead to penetration into dentine, thus making a restoration obligatory.

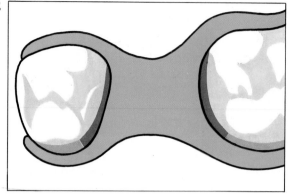

372 The required location of a guide surface will be dependent on its function: the guide surface (red) will be needed on the proximal surface of the abutment tooth facing the edentulous space to control the path of insertion of the saddle; to reciprocate the retentive clasp, the guide surface (green) should be on the tooth surface diametrically opposite the retentive portion of the clasp.

Unfavourable survey lines

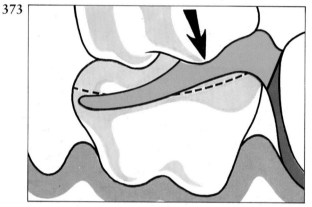

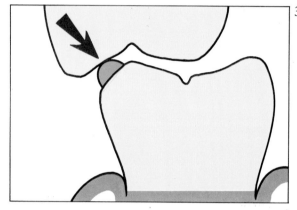

373 and 374 A high survey line on a tooth which is to be clasped is unfavourable because it requires the clasp to be placed too close to the occlusal surface and may create an occlusal interference (arrows).

Even if an occlusal interference is not present a high clasp arm is more noticeable to the patient and may interfere with mastication.

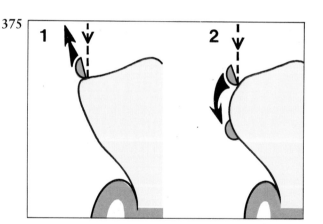

375 (1) A high survey line may also result in deformation of the clasp because, on insertion, the clasp is prevented from moving down the tooth by contact with the occlusal surface. If the patient persists in trying to seat the denture, the clasp is bent upwards rather than flexed outwards.

(2) Shaping the enamel to lower the survey line will allow the clasp to be positioned further gingivally and it also provides a 'lead-in' during insertion, causing the clasp to flex outwards over the survey line as planned.

Retentive areas

376 Retentive areas can be created by grinding enamel. However, the enamel is relatively thin in the gingival third of the crown where the retentive tip of the clasp would normally be placed, so the amount of undercut that can be achieved by these means without penetrating the enamel is strictly limited. It is usually better to establish improved contours for retention by restorative methods as outlined in Chapter 20.

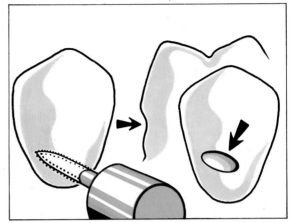

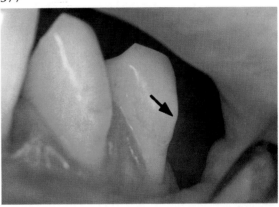

377 Undercut areas can also be created by the use of acid-etch composite restorations.

A broad area of attachment of the restoration to the enamel is desirable as this will reduce the chance of the restoration being displaced and will produce a contour more suitable for clasping.

Conventional composites should not be used for this purpose as they can cause marked abrasion of the clasp arm with consequent weakening of the clasp and loss of retention. In order to minimise the mutual abrasion of composite and clasp, ultra-fine composite and a more flexible design of clasp should be selected.

Part 4
Prosthetic treatment

In this part we consider the clinical procedures involved in the construction of partial dentures. The various chapters offer a basic guide to these procedures as we believe that the details of technique can be appreciated only by clinical tuition and experience.

22 Working impressions

Working impressions are obtained after the denture has been designed and any tooth preparation completed. It should be remembered that even in the absence of obvious mucosal injury an existing denture will have had a significant influence on the form of the denture-bearing mucosa. Recovery of the mucosa after removal of the denture can take several hours. Therefore a patient should be advised to leave the denture out for at least four hours before attending for the working impression. There will of course be some patients who are unable to comply with this advice for social reasons.

Individual tray

The production of a working cast sufficiently accurate for the construction of a partial denture frequently necessitates the use of an individual tray. Such a tray enables an accurate impression to be made of the functional depth and width of the sulci in those areas which will be related to the denture border and to components such as gingivally approaching clasps, connecting bars and plates.

378 In order to produce an accurate impression the tray should be constructed so that it is uniformly spaced from the teeth and adjacent tissues. This will provide for the even layer of impression material of sufficient thickness necessary for optimum elastic recovery on removal from the mouth.

378

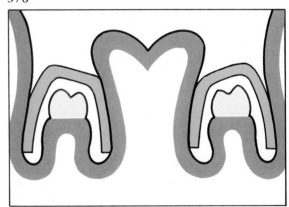

379

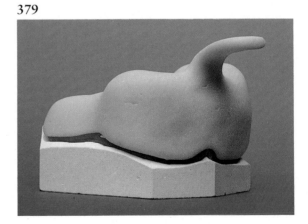

379 Individual trays are usually made from cold-curing acrylic resin with a high filler content. The tray material is accurately moulded over a wax spacer of 3 mm thickness. The borders are trimmed until they are smooth and located uniformly 2 mm short of the depth of the sulci to allow for unrestricted movement of the adjacent tissues.

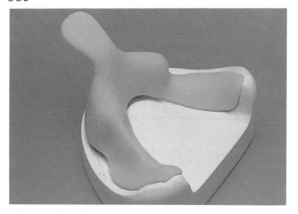

380 Rigidity of the tray is important. Therefore, where the 'U' cross-sectional shape is lacking, as may occur in resorbed edentulous areas, the tray should be stiffened by the addition to its external surface of a fin of acrylic tray material as on the left hand side of this lower tray. The fin has the additional benefit of providing a finger rest while the tray is held in position to record the impression.

After construction, the tray must be set aside for about 10 hours to reach a stable state. If used immediately, the stresses built into the tray during the moulding of the material will still be undergoing relief, thus reducing the accuracy of the impression.

The use of stops

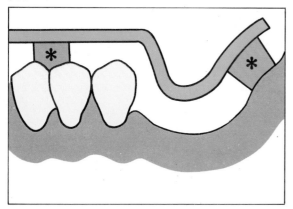

381 Before any attempt is made at the chairside to adjust the border of the tray, it is recommended that impression compound be added to selected areas of the internal surface of the tray in order to form stops.

Stops re-establish the intended spacing and permit the accurate relocation of the tray every time it is inserted into the mouth, thus allowing the borders to be trimmed to their correct position in relation to the functional depth of the sulci.

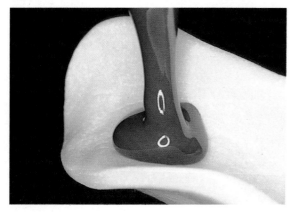

382 Stops are formed by softening the end of a stick of impression compound and by applying it to the chosen location on the tray. The compound is then flamed and tempered in warm water and the tray located in the mouth under gentle pressure, thus moulding the stops to a thickness of approximately 3 mm.

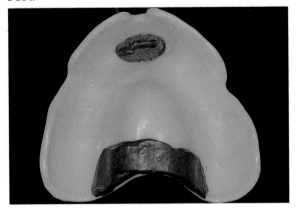

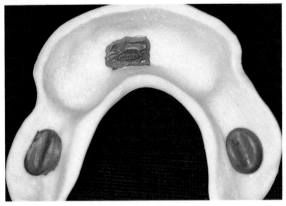

383a and 383b For optimum effectiveness the stops must be carefully positioned to ensure 3-point location of the tray. Suitable locations for stops include those areas related to the incisal or occlusal surfaces of the teeth, the palatal vault and posterior border, and the retromolar pads. They should not be placed over teeth that are to be covered by denture components as the shape of these teeth should be recorded by an optimum thickness of impression material. Any stops that include more than the incisal edges or cusp tips should be reduced as the excess material may hinder reseating of the tray.

384

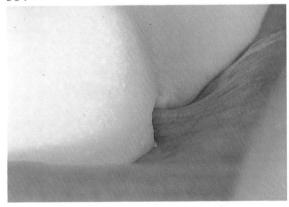

384 Once the stops have been completed, the tray is reinserted into the mouth. Gentle retraction of the lips and cheeks will indicate labial or buccal over- or underextension. Any areas of over-extension should be reduced, as here where space has been created for the buccal fraenum. Any areas of underextension should be made good by the addition of a border moulding material such as tracing compound. For free-end saddles the tray should cover the retromolar pads or enclose the tuberosities.

385

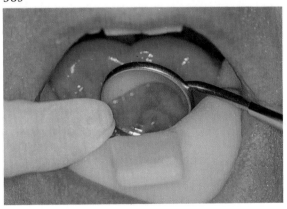

385 Assessment of the lingual extension of the lower tray is difficult because of the mobility of the sulcus tissues and poor visibility. Anteriorly, the extension can be checked with the aid of a mouth mirror and posteriorly by the diagnostic addition of tracing compound to the tray.

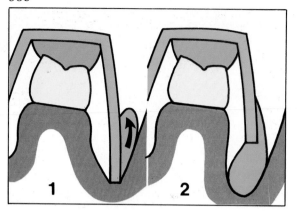

386 Lingual border moulding is carried out by asking the patient to raise the tongue to contact the upper lip and then to touch each corner of the mouth in turn. If the added material is totally displaced from the edge of the tray by tongue movements (1) the overextended border must be reduced; if the compound has been moulded to form an extension of the lower border (2) it is chilled and left in place.

Choice of impression material

Alginate of a low viscosity is suitable providing that none of the undercuts is so great that the material is stressed beyond its elastic limit

when the impression is withdrawn from the mouth.

387

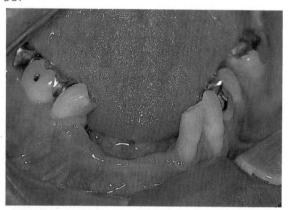

387 Here, bilateral lingually tilted premolars create severe undercuts and it is advisable to choose an elastomeric material such as silicone, polysulphide or polyether. All these materials possess superior elastic recovery compared with alginate.

The appropriate adhesive for the chosen material must be applied to the tray in a uniformly thin layer. It is most important that the adhesive film be allowed to dry before the impression material is brought into contact with it.

388

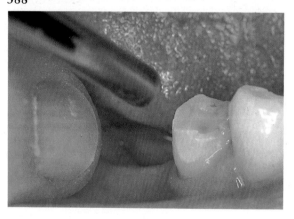

Preparation of the mouth

388 The layer of saliva that would otherwise hinder the flow of impression material into direct contact with the teeth should be removed using a warm air syringe. This is particularly indicated when there are depressions in the tooth surface, such as rest seat preparations, and where silicone impression materials are to be used. However, excessive drying should be avoided, otherwise direct adherence of the impression material to the tissues may occur.

389 Open interdental spaces should be occluded with soft wax prior to inserting the loaded impression tray, otherwise the impression material will flow beneath the contact points and lock the impression in place. Removal of the impression would thus result in distortion. The wax should obviously not be permitted to stray on to a tooth surface that is to be contacted by any denture component.

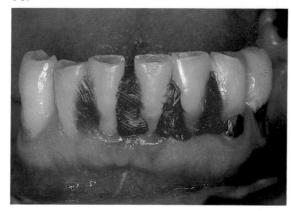

Completing the impression

For maximum accuracy, the impression material must be thoroughly mixed, the tray loaded, inserted and seated in the mouth and border moulding completed before the working time of the material has elapsed. It is difficult to determine clinically when the working time of an elastomer has been reached, since the viscosity of these materials begins to increase immediately mixing is commenced. Thus the working time as stated by the manufacturer of the material must be observed.

390 It is helpful if alginate impression material is wiped over the teeth and into deep sulci with a finger immediately prior to inserting the loaded tray. Air is thereby displaced from these areas ensuring an impression free from airblows.

The tray should not be loaded with excessive quantities of material, since there should be only 3 mm between an accurately adjusted tray and the oral tissues. Excess material may flow and embarrass the patient's airway or hinder accurate seating of the tray and moulding of the borders of the impression.

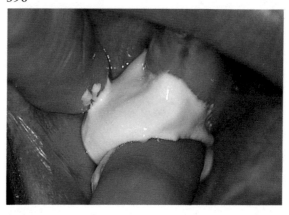

The loaded tray should be seated on its stops, border moulding completed, and then held with only sufficient pressure to keep it in position. Continued pressure, with or without inadvertent movement of the tray, may introduce stresses into the setting impression material and may deform the tray and the oral structures that support it.

Once the manufacturer's stated setting time has been reached, snap removal of the completed impression is effected. Saliva is rinsed from the impression which is then inspected for accuracy.

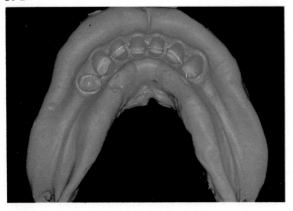

391 A good impression should have rounded borders that are correctly supported by the tray. There should be a minimum of airblows, which should be entirely absent from areas that are to be contacted by any part of the metal framework. Ideally, no portion of the tray (except for the stops) should show through the impression.

392

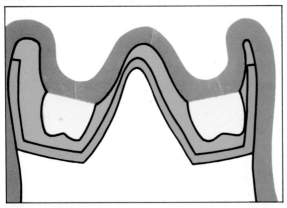

392 Gross asymmetry of the width of the sulci may indicate that the tray was not correctly centred in the mouth and was not seated on the stops. Such errors of positioning frequently result in the complete displacement of impression material from some areas of the tray.

393

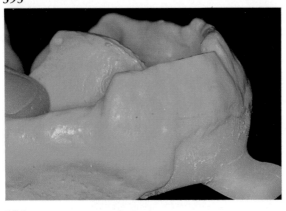

393 and 394 Common faults are underextension of the tray borders or incomplete seating of the tray on its stops. Both faults lead to inadequate support for the impression material. The correct depth and width of the sulci are unlikely to have been recorded and the impression material is almost certain to be distorted when pouring the cast.

394

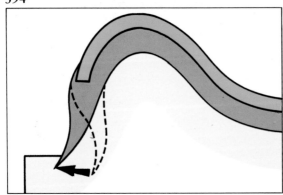

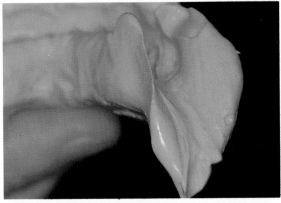

395 Particularly vulnerable in this respect is the lingual pouch. The impression material is unlikely to record the functional depth and width of the sulcus unless the tray is correctly extended and seated. The sharp border seen here indicates inadequate tray extension.

396

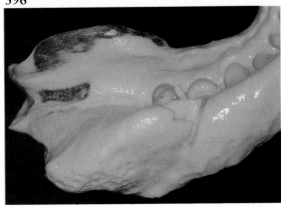

396 If the border of the tray was overextended the true functional form of the sulci may not have been recorded. Such overextension should be reduced and the impression retaken.

If the impression needs to be retaken, all the set impression material must be removed from the tray, and another thin layer of adhesive applied and allowed to dry before the new attempt is made. Multiple retakes may result in a thick layer of adhesive on the tray. Such a layer exhibits poor adhesive properties; it must therefore be removed before a new thin layer is applied.

397 Care must be taken to preserve the functional depth and width of the sulci recorded with the impression. It is difficult to attach wax beading to alginate and elastomer impression materials; however, an indelible pencil can be used to draw a line on the outside of the impression 3 mm away from the border.

Once accepted, the impression may be immersed in a disinfectant, rinsed and then cast as soon as possible. In the interim period, alginate materials should be stored under conditions of 100 per cent humidity (**107**). Elastomers should be stored dry in sealable plastic bags. As with preliminary impressions, precautions must be taken to prevent pressure deformation of the impression material.

397

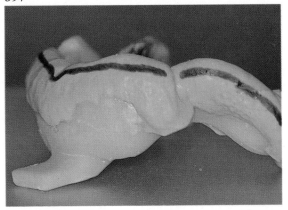

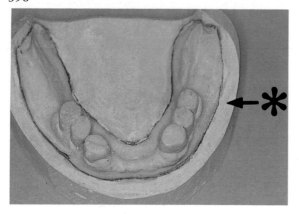

398 Trimming of the cast should be stopped once the pencil mark on the stone is reached. An adequate area of 'land' * is thus created on the cast.

399

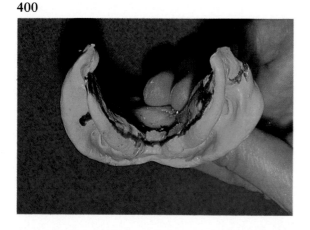

Impression procedure for sub-lingual bars

399 (1) If this connector is not to interfere with tongue movements, a very careful record must be made of the functional depth and width of the lingual sulcus throughout the extent of the connector. The tray should be so formed that the lingual border is spaced only 1mm from the alveolar mucosa in order to avoid distorting the functional width of the sulcus. To prevent inadvertent contact between this periphery and the alveolar mucosa, it is essential to employ correctly positioned stops.

(2) The periphery may now be refined by using a border moulding material such as tracing compound. This material should be of sufficiently low viscosity to avoid distension of the sulcus.

The material is moulded by requesting the patient to move the tip of the tongue from one corner of the mouth to the other, following the contour of the upper lip.

400

400 The impression is completed with the aid of a fairly low viscosity material. While the material is setting, the patient is requested to repeat the tongue movements. After removal, the impression of the lingual sulcus must be carefully inspected. The border moulding material should be covered by a thin wash of impression material. When satisfied as to the accuracy of the impression, the clinician should demarcate the depth and width of the lingual sulcus with an indelible pencil line.

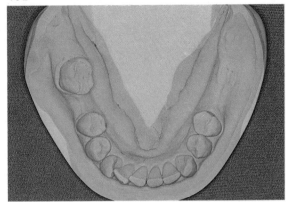

401 The technician must then take care when pouring the impression and trimming the cast to ensure that the functional depth and width of the sulcus so carefully recorded is preserved.

The impressions should be sent to the laboratory together with appropriate instructions for the work to be completed for the next clinical stage. If a metal framework is required, the design is indicated on the prescription sheet or study cast. The framework may incorporate an acrylic resin tray for the altered cast technique (Chapter 25). Occlusal rims may be constructed on appropriate bases. If a wax trial denture is required, details of tooth shade, mould and position will have to be supplied.

23 Recording the jaw relationship

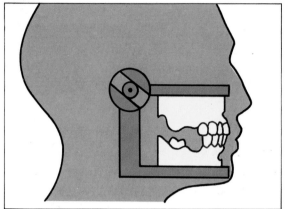

Objective

402 The objective of this stage of clinical treatment is to record a specific jaw relationship, such as the intercuspal position or the retruded position, so that the casts can be mounted on an articulator, thus permitting correct positioning of the artificial teeth.

The degree of complexity of the task is related to the number and occlusal relationship of the remaining teeth and may be categorised as follows.

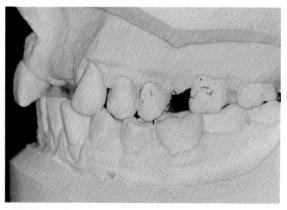

403 Sufficient teeth may be present to enable the casts to be placed together accurately in a stable intercuspal position at the desired vertical and horizontal jaw relationship. Thus no additional visit by the patient is required to record the jaw relationship.

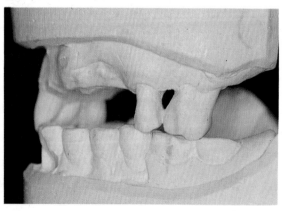

404 Often the desired jaw relationship cannot be so easily reproduced outside the mouth even in the presence of an occlusal stop because there may be insufficient occluding teeth to produce a stable position of the casts.

405 Alternatively, the occlusal stop may produce an intercuspal position at an unacceptable horizontal and vertical jaw relationship. Tilting or drifting of teeth or loss of tooth substance by abrasion, attrition or erosion may be contributory factors resulting in mandibular deviation or reduced occlusal vertical dimension.

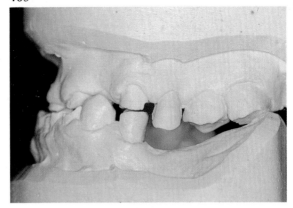

406 Frequently the remaining teeth are so placed in the jaws that they do not provide even an occlusal stop, let alone a stable cast relationship.

For these last three situations, occlusal rims are adjusted in the mouth to record the desired jaw relationship so that it can be transferred to the casts.

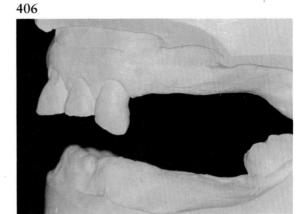

407 The wax occlusal rims may be placed on temporary bases of shellac or acrylic resin, or on the definitive cast metal frameworks. These must be tried in the mouth and their stability checked. If the stability is poor, yet the baseplate fits the cast accurately, consideration must be given to the possibility that the problem is due to an inaccurate impression. If this is confirmed the working impression must be retaken. The retention of the occlusal rim must be sufficient to maintain the rim in position during subsequent recording procedures.

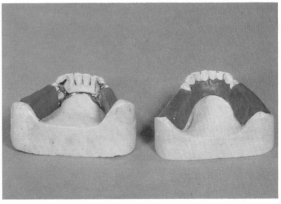

Adjustment of the rims

Occlusal rims should only be placed in the mouth long enough to carry out a particular clinical procedure. They must then be removed immediately and chilled in a bowl of cold water to prevent distortion.

If an anterior saddle replaces only one or two teeth, there will be sufficient guidance from the remaining teeth to determine the position of the artificial replacements.

408

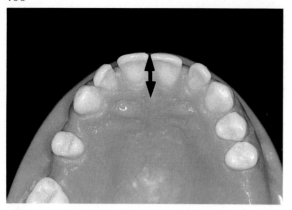

408 When maxillary anterior teeth are present, the mid-incisal point will generally be located about 1 cm in front of the centre of the incisive papilla. If teeth are missing, this relationship is a useful guide when trimming the labial surface of a rim in order to restore the appearance and provide the appropriate lip support.

409

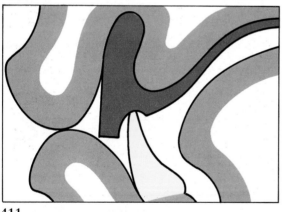

409 The anterior inferior border of the rim should be adjusted to indicate the desired incisal level. This is decided by reference to any adjacent teeth and to the resting level of the upper lip. A line may also be scribed on the labial face of the rim to indicate the projected midline of the incisors.

Where many anterior teeth are missing the rim should be carved until its incisal level is parallel to the imaginary horizontal line joining the pupils of the eyes (interpupillary line).

410

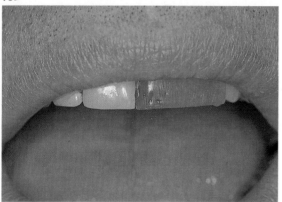

410 To achieve the correct jaw relationship when an edentulous area in the upper anterior region is opposed by natural lower anterior teeth, the upper rim may require to be thinned from the palatal aspect to accommodate these teeth. The inferior border and labial face of the upper anterior wax rim should be preserved to indicate the desired position of the artificial teeth.

The upper wax rims in any posterior edentulous areas are trimmed until they indicate the desired position of the occlusal plane.

411

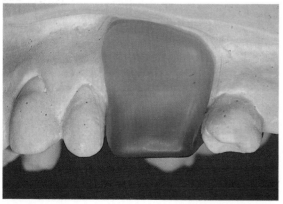

411 Sufficient posterior teeth may be present to indicate the approximate level of the occlusal plane.

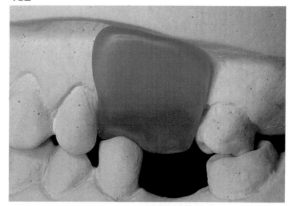

412 Where opposing natural teeth are present these will normally be the determining factor in finalising the position of the occlusal surface of the rim. Here the rim has been modified to accommodate a lower tooth that has erupted beyond the projected occlusal plane.

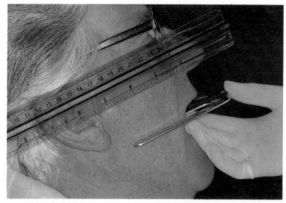

413 If many posterior teeth are missing, the upper rim should be carved until it is parallel to the line joining the inferior border of the ala of the nose to the midpoint of the tragus of the ear with the aid, if desired, of an occlusal plane guide.

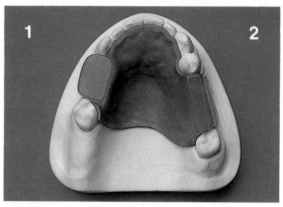

414 The width of the rim should also be adjusted until it indicates the desired buccolingual positioning of the teeth. The rim (1) is too bulky, whilst rim (2) has been corrected.

In the absence of a posterior abutment tooth to act as a guide, the buccal side of the upper rim should just contact the cheek mucosa when the mouth is half open.

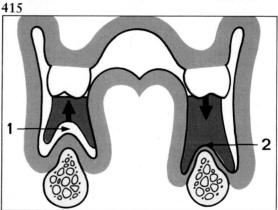

415 The lower occlusal rim is inserted and adjusted until it meets the upper rim or teeth evenly under minimal pressure in the desired jaw relationship. The rim should not then tilt away from the denture bearing mucosa (1) or compress the mucosa or the wax of the rim (2). Tilting or compression will result in the casts not being articulated in the same relationship as the patient's jaws.

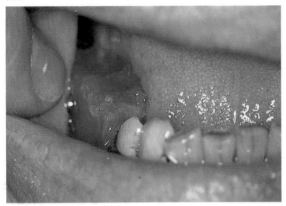

416 The lower rim is also adjusted until it indicates the position of the teeth in the neutral zone. This rim is encroaching on the tongue space and needs to be reduced on its lingual aspect.

 417

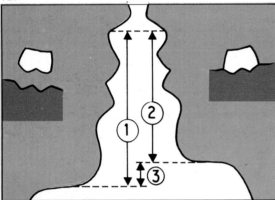

417 The jaw relationship may be indicated by intercuspation of some of the remaining teeth. Where the existing jaw relationship is not acceptable or there is no positive occlusal stop, the resting vertical dimension (1) should be assessed. The occlusal vertical dimension of the rims (2) must then be adjusted so that an adequate freeway space (3) is provided.

When guidance from posterior teeth has been lost, the jaw relationship in the horizontal plane should be recorded with the mandible in the retruded position, which is readily reproducible.

Finalising the registration with an acceptable occlusal stop

418

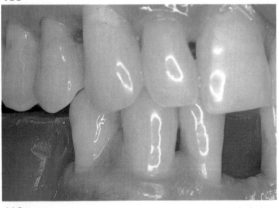

418 A further millimetre of wax is removed from the occlusal surface of the rims to provide a slight gap between opposing rims or teeth, thus avoiding the possibility of occlusal pressure distorting either wax or mucosa. To permit subsequent separation of the occlusal rims, one of the rims (usually the upper) and its associated teeth are lightly coated with petroleum jelly.

419

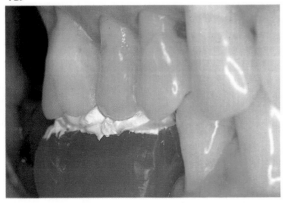

419 The space between the rims is then taken up by a recording medium that should be of uniformly low viscosity (to avoid wax/mucosa compression) and should set rigidly (to prevent subsequent loss of the accurate registration). Impression plaster or a modified zinc oxide/eugenol paste fulfils these conditions; the commonly used softened wax does not.

Finalising the registration without an acceptable occlusal stop

Once the correct occlusal vertical dimension has been achieved, no more wax is removed from the rims. If this were done the occlusal vertical dimension would be decreased; otherwise the registration procedure is as above.

Checking the registration

420 Any recording medium that has flowed beyond the tips of the opposing cusps or edge of the opposing rims is carefully trimmed so that only shallow indentations remain. This aids direct visual assessment of the accuracy of the record in the mouth.

421 The casts are now placed in occlusion using the occlusal rims. Trimming of the casts may be necessary to permit accurate assembly, since their heels may touch each other or portions of the opposing rim or baseplate.

The patient must close into the retruded jaw relationship and maintain that position while the recording medium sets under minimal pressure.

420

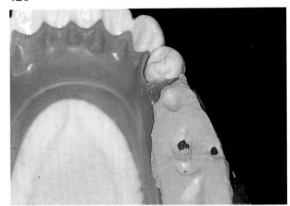

421

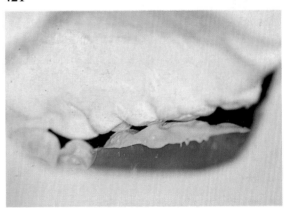

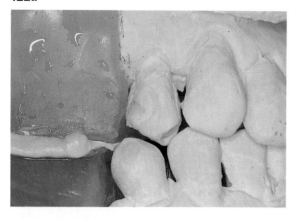

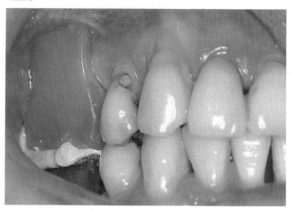

422a and **422b** Above all, it is important to remember that it is the clinician's responsibility to ensure that the desired jaw relationship has been transferred accurately from the mouth to the casts.

The relationship of the natural teeth to each other must thus be inspected; if they are further apart on the casts than they are in the mouth, compression of the wax or mucosa must be suspected.

Information for the laboratory

The following information must be written on the laboratory prescription sheet:

1 The unwanted undercuts that need to be blocked out on the cast.
2 The shade, mould and material to be used for the artificial teeth.
3 The desired arrangement (rotation, inclination, spacing, etc.) of any anterior teeth.

4 The type of articulator that is to be used. When a semi-adjustable articulator is required, the laboratory should be supplied with the necessary facebow and occlusal records (Chapter 6).

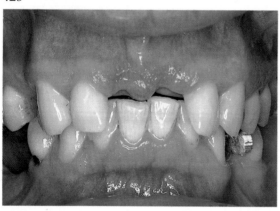

423 and **424** When metal backings are required for the artificial anterior teeth, as might be the case when opposing natural teeth are virtually contacting the mucosa of the edentulous area, a request should be made for a wax trial insertion of the teeth

on a shellac or acrylic resin baseplate to be provided before the metal framework is constructed. This is because the definitive position of the artificial teeth must be decided before the metal is cast.

24 Trial insertion of the metal framework

It is recommended that the trial insertion of the metal framework should initially be undertaken without the addition of any wax rims or artificial teeth. If the casting does not fit into place at once, the presence of wax hinders the search for interferences and additionally, if the casting needs adjustment with stones, the

heat generated may melt the wax.

If desired, the framework in a free-end edentulous area may have a close fitting temporary acrylic resin base attached to it to permit the recording of an altered cast impression (Chapter 25).

425 The framework is first examined on the cast to ensure that the prescribed design has been followed. Any wrought components should have been included and attached to the cast-metal framework by solder or cold-curing acrylic resin. All components should be checked to ensure that the fit is accurate, that they are of adequate dimensions and are correctly positioned.

425

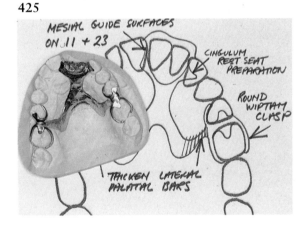

426

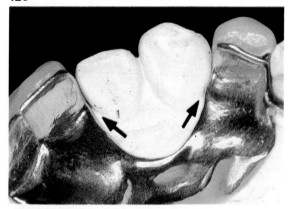

426 to **428** These components are not correctly positioned, being too close to the gingival margins or failing to cross the margins at an angle of at least 90°.

427

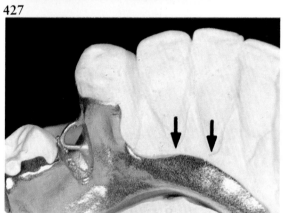

428

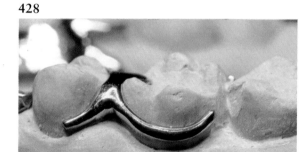

429

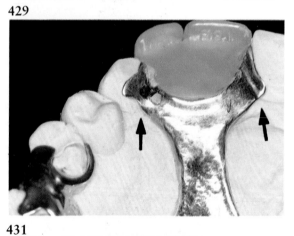

430

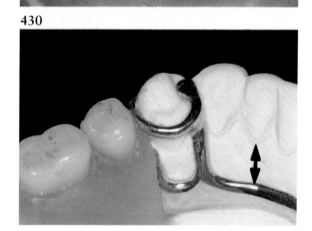

429 to **431** Correct positioning.

431

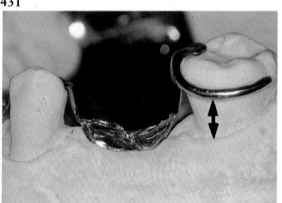

432 The stability of the casting should be checked under finger pressure. Kennedy Class I and II frameworks with a spaced mesh will rock if pressure is applied to the saddle area unless a stop or foot (arrowed) is provided to support the mesh. Fully tooth-supported frameworks should not rock.

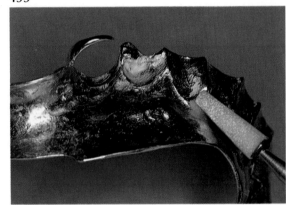

433 The fitting surface of major connectors covering the gingival margin should be inspected. Any sharp metal entering the gingival crevice should be removed. This must be done with care, however, as excessive stoning will create a space beneath the connector into which the gingivae will proliferate (**269**).

The framework is now tried in the mouth, utilising the intended path of insertion.

If the framework does not seat fully, no attempt should be made to force it into place as subsequent removal from the mouth may be extremely difficult. A systematic search must be undertaken to discover what is preventing complete seating. Any areas of abrasion on the cast may indicate the location of inaccuracies in the framework. Clinical examination with a mouth mirror may reveal interfering contacts between framework and teeth. Gentle rocking of the framework may reveal a discrepancy of fit acting as a fulcrum.

434 More precise location of any interference may be achieved by the use of disclosing aids such as this soft wax which is melted and then flowed on to the suspect area of the framework, which is seated as far as it will go, and then withdrawn. Initial contacts between the framework and teeth will be visible as areas where the disclosing wax has been displaced, exposing the metal. These contacts can then be eliminated.

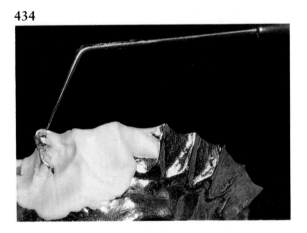

435 Care must be taken to avoid damaging those portions of connectors that are occlusal to the survey lines, otherwise a space is created between denture and tooth surface into which food can pack. Anything other than relatively minor adjustments to the framework indicates a generally poor fit, and consideration must be given to retaking the master impression and obtaining a new framework.

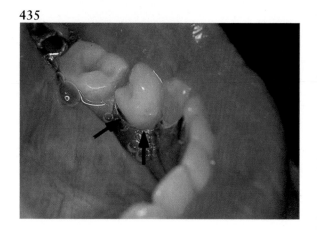

435

Once the framework is seated in the mouth, its stability is assessed. A decision as to whether an altered cast impression will be taken must be made before the jaw relationship is recorded.

The fit and positioning of all the component parts of the framework are again assessed, including the extension of the mandibular major connector in relation to the functional depth of the sulcus. If unsatisfactory, a new impression and casting are required.

436 When natural teeth are being utilised to provide an occlusal stop, care should be taken to check that the framework does not alter this occlusal relationship. The patient's comments are valuable in detecting the presence and location of occlusal prematurities. Such comments must be supplemented by visual assessment, by the use of articulating paper to mark occlusal contacts and by testing the ability of the teeth to grip a strip of thin metal foil (shimstock). Premature occlusal contacts must be eliminated by selective grinding until the desired jaw relationship is established.

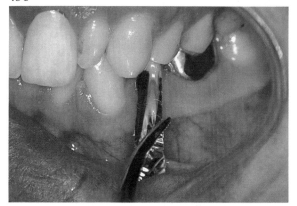

436

The laboratory should be requested to set up the teeth on the framework, as indicated at the conclusion of Chapter 23, ready for the trial insertion of the waxed-up denture.

25 Altered cast technique

437 When a free-end saddle is constructed on a cast poured from a mucostatic impression, the differential in the support offered by the abutment tooth in its relatively incompressible periodontal ligament and the more compressible denture-bearing mucosa is greatest. As a result, the tendency for the free-end saddle to sink under occlusal load and pivot about the rest on the abutment tooth is increased.

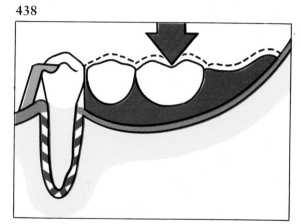

438 The objective of the altered cast technique is to reduce the support differential for a free-end saddle by obtaining a compressive impression of the edentulous area under conditions which mimic functional loading. The distribution of load from the denture to the residual ridge is thus improved and the denture is more stable.

439 Acrylic resin tray material is added to the framework to form a base which covers the relevant edentulous area. It must be of sufficient thickness to be rigid. At the chairside the periphery of the base is inspected for under- or overextension and adjusted accordingly. Any undercuts in the impression surface are removed. This surface is dried and zinc oxide impression paste or medium viscosity silicone impression material applied.

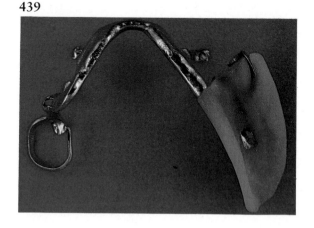

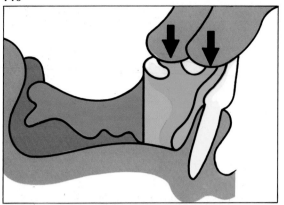

440 The framework is placed in the mouth and great care must be taken to ensure that it is seated on the teeth by pressure on the occlusal rests and indirect retainers *only* – no finger pressure is applied to the base area and the teeth are not occluded. Once the framework is fully seated, border moulding is carried out.

441

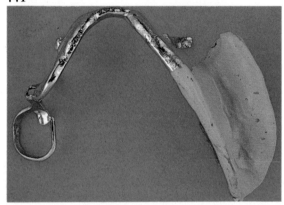

441 When the impression material has set, the framework is removed from the mouth and the impression inspected. Any errors must be corrected by appropriate modification or by retaking the impression.

In the original approach to the altered cast technique the impression is developed using a specially formulated wax which flows readily at mouth temperature. This technique has the advantage of allowing progressive modification of the impression until an ideal result is achieved. However, it requires significantly more chairside time than the technique described and employs a commercial wax (Korrecta Wax No. 4 (Kerr)) that is not readily obtainable, or a mixture of waxes (75 per cent paraffin wax, 25 per cent yellow beeswax) that needs to be specifically prepared.

442

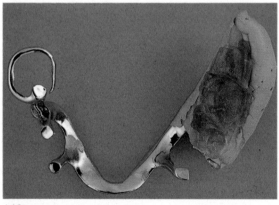

442 Once a satisfactory impression has been obtained the need for an extra clinical stage to record the jaw relationship can be avoided by adding wax rims to the framework at the chairside and proceeding with the recording at the same appointment.

443

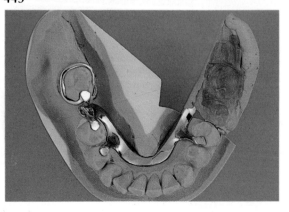

443 When the completed impression has been conveyed to the laboratory, the relevant edentulous areas are cut from the original master cast. The framework is carefully and accurately seated on the teeth.

444 Finally, a new composite cast is produced by pouring artificial stone into the saddle impression.

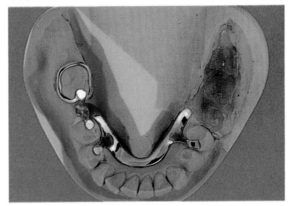

444

An alternative procedure involves rebasing the completed denture. Zinc oxide impression paste is applied to the acrylic fitting surface of the relevant saddles, and an impression taken with the denture being seated by pressure on the occlusal rests and indirect retainers only. Pressure is not applied to the occlusal surfaces of the artificial teeth. The resulting impression is used to rebase the saddle.

445 A disadvantage of this method is that it will usually disrupt the evenness of occlusal contact in the saddle area by creating premature contacts posteriorly. The occlusal correction required can be quite considerable.

445

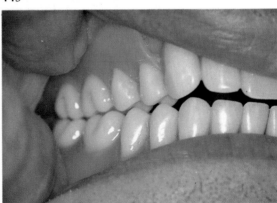

26 Trial insertion of waxed-up dentures

This is the last stage at which modifications can be made before the wax is replaced by acrylic. A careful routine must be followed to prevent any errors from continuing through to the finished dentures.

Wax try-in for metal dentures

Each denture should first be examined on the articulated casts.

446 The positioning of any posterior teeth is compared with the position of the remaining natural teeth and with the prescription supplied to the laboratory via the occlusal rim if this is available. For example, teeth on bounded saddles (e.g. **25** and **26**) should be in line with the buccal surfaces of the natural teeth. Palatally placed teeth (e.g. **15** and **14**) will encroach on the space for the tongue. Tooth positions will need to be confirmed on intraoral examination.

446

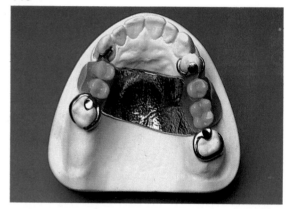

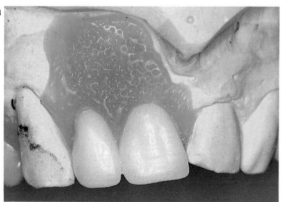

447a and **447b** The arrangement of the anterior teeth should be pleasing to the eye and conform to any requests on the laboratory card. The labial surfaces and incisal edges should harmonise with the abutment teeth. If incisal wear is present on the natural teeth it should be simulated on the denture.

The appearance of the incisors in (**a**) is less acceptable than that in (**b**). The appearance may need to be modified after both the patient and dentist have had the opportunity to view the denture in the mouth.

The intercuspation of the teeth should be even and, in order to reduce the magnitude of the potentially damaging lateral forces, as much balanced occlusion and articulation as possible should be provided within the constraints imposed by the remaining natural teeth. Guidance should, wherever possible, be provided by the natural teeth.

448 Wax flanges should be of a thickness and extension corresponding to the amount of bone resorption in the area so that they only replace the tissue that has been lost and restore the former contour of the alveolar ridge. Mesial and distal borders should be thin so that the flange blends with the adjacent mucosa, thus avoiding food trapping and promoting patient comfort.

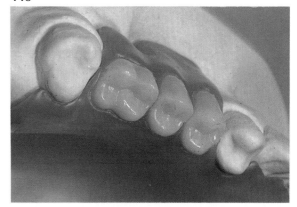

448

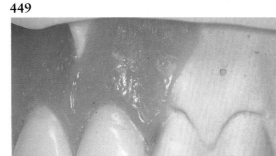

449

449 If the path of insertion and withdrawal permits, the lateral borders of any anterior flange should be thinned and should terminate over the convexities produced by the roots of the abutment teeth. This arrangement should also permit the labial flange to restore the papilla of the abutment tooth next to the edentulous space. The positioning and contour of papillae and gingival margins around the artificial teeth should harmonise with those of the adjacent natural teeth.

450a

450b

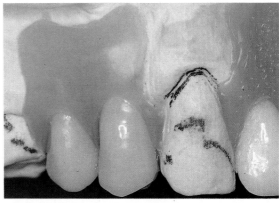

450a and **450b** A common error, which creates a poor appearance, is to place the gum margin of the artificial upper premolars at a much lower level than that of the adjacent natural teeth (**a**). This may be overcome by careful waxing up and by the selection of an artificial tooth of appropriate crown length (**b**).

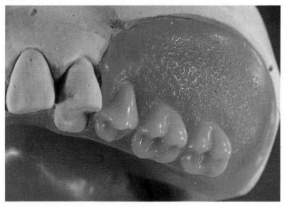

451 The borders of mucosa- or partially mucosa-supported saddles should extend to the full depth of the sulci recorded on the cast in order that the occlusal forces may be distributed as widely as possible and that the adjacent musculature may be utilised to reinforce the retention and stability of the prosthesis.

452

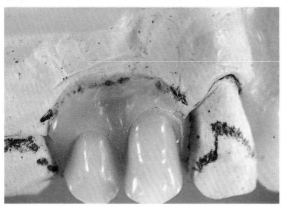

452 If the chosen path of insertion and withdrawal for the denture does not eliminate undercuts on the labial or buccal sides of the ridge, the flanges should be thinned as they pass over the survey line and end approximately 1 mm beyond it.

The dentures are now seated in the mouth along their planned path of insertion and the fit, positioning of all components and flange extension are checked by visual inspection. Functional movements of the lips, cheeks and tongue should not displace the denture. The relationship of the artificial teeth to the soft tissues should be assessed to determine whether the prescription supplied by the occlusal rims has been followed. The vertical and horizontal jaw relationships are checked utilising the patient's comments, visual assessment and shimstock. If natural teeth provide an acceptable occlusal stop it is important to ensure that these and the artificial teeth are in even contact. If natural teeth are not determining the jaw relationship, it is important to ensure that there is even contact in the retruded jaw relationship at the desired occlusal vertical dimension.

453

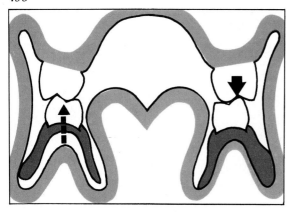

453 The patient must maintain only the lightest possible occlusal contact while the occlusion is being checked, otherwise any premature occlusal contact may be masked by distortion of the denture base, by displacement of the mucosa or, as shown here, by movement of the trial denture away from the tissues.

Correction of significant occlusal errors will require the replacement of the artificial teeth with wax rims so that the jaw relationship can be re-recorded.

454 The shade, mould and arrangement of the artificial teeth should harmonise with the natural teeth.

The incisal edges of the natural anterior teeth tend to follow the curve formed by the lower lip when smiling. Reproduction of this relationship when positioning artificial anterior teeth can contribute significantly to a pleasing appearance.

The patient may be able to recall distinguishing features of the missing natural teeth or may be in possession of suitable photographs. Remember that a totally regular arrangement of artificial teeth almost always looks artificial.

455 On occasion, seemingly bizarre requests from the patient may be accepted, provided that they do not compromise the stability, retention and function of the denture. If the request is not met, the denture may be totally rejected by the patient. Indeed, tooth arrangements that appear exaggerated out of the mouth are often acceptable *in vivo* as seen on this completed denture.

456 The smooth surface of the flange shown here should be avoided if the flange is likely to be visible during function as it produces an artificial appearance. Instead, the flange should be stippled and contoured to mimic the mucosal surface and break up reflected light in a more natural manner.

The unsatisfactory appearance is also due to the difference in shade between 11 and 21 and to the slight discrepancy in the incisal level.

457 Any stains to be incorporated in the teeth or acrylic resin flange should be indicated on a drawing attached to the laboratory prescription card.

454

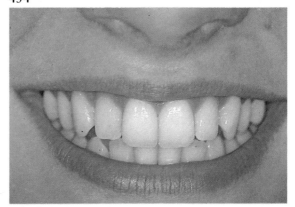

455

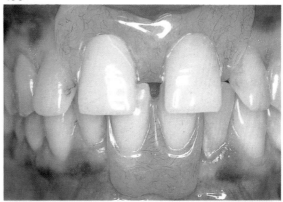

456

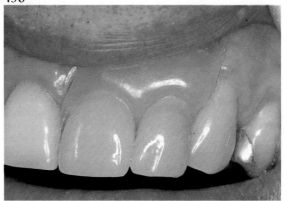

457

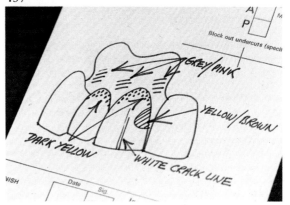

458

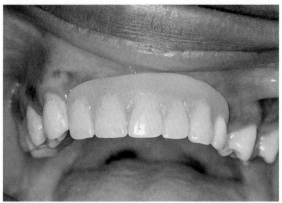

458 These instructions are particularly important where there is pigmentation of the mucosa. Failure to tint the flange to match the adjacent mucosa will result in the highly unsatisfactory appearance shown here.

459

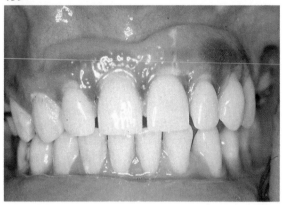

459 Carefully planned and executed tinting of the labial flange can create this convincingly natural result.

The appearance of the trial denture must always be discussed with the patient, using a mirror (preferably wall-mounted to ensure that viewing takes place at conversation distance) to view the situation before and after any modification. Approval of the appearance must be obtained before the denture is processed.

460

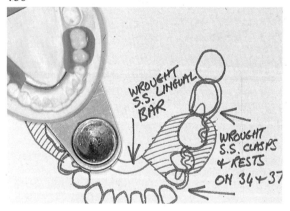

Wax try-in for acrylic dentures

Each denture should first be examined on the articulated casts.

460 The designs should be checked against the prescription supplied to the laboratory. Wrought rests and clasps should be omitted at this stage as they cannot be securely attached to the connector. They are therefore liable to move during the trial insertion of the denture and their contribution to retention and stability cannot be assessed.

461 In situations where the gingival margin is to be left uncovered, the border of the trial denture is examined to ensure that it is at least 3 mm clear of the gingival margins, and that where it crosses the margins it does so at 90° or more (1). It may be difficult to achieve this amount of clearance in relation to lone standing teeth such as 13 and it may therefore be more appropriate to cover the palatal gingival margin (2).

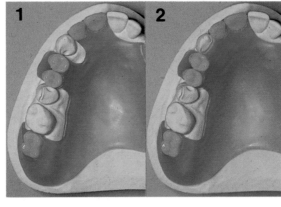

462 Where the wax contacts natural teeth, it must do so at or above the survey lines *. If it ends below the line, a gap between acrylic and tooth will result when the completed denture is inserted which would permit denture movement and food packing. Where the tooth surface is not undercut, relief should not be provided for the gingival margins.

The positioning of the teeth, the contouring of the wax flanges and stability of the denture on the cast are checked as described previously.

462

463 It is important to ensure that unwanted undercuts have been blocked out as requested on the laboratory card. If, as in the illustration, wax has been used for this purpose, the cast must be duplicated prior to the processing of the denture.

463

The dentures are now seated in the mouth along their planned paths of insertion. Fit and stability are carefully assessed. Allowance must be made for the inexact fit of the baseplate. The flange extension is checked and appropriate corrective measures undertaken.

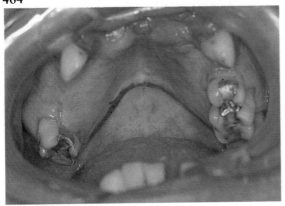

464 When an acrylic connector is to be fully extended posteriorly, it should terminate just anterior to the line where movement of the soft palate begins (here marked with indelible pencil). A groove, the post-dam, is cut into the cast in this position, extending through each hamular notch. The depth and width of the groove depends on the tissue compressibility as determined by palpation; the groove being generally deeper and wider laterally in the palate than in the midline.

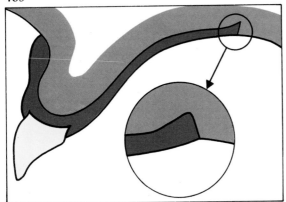

465 The post-dam has a vertical posterior wall and is chamfered anteriorly. This permits the posterior border of the plate to be thinned and turned into the tissues, adding to patient comfort and creating a posterior seal.

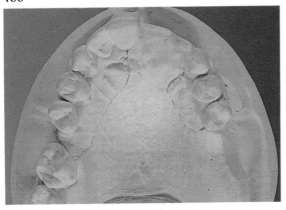

466 Narrower grooves, their depth again determined by clinical assessment of tissue compressibility, are also cut into the mucosal areas of the cast along the other proposed borders of palatal acrylic connectors. These 'pin-dams' produce close adaptation of the borders, reducing the ingress of food.

The positioning of the posterior teeth, the jaw relationships, and the appearance are checked as described previously.

Instructions to the laboratory

The laboratory card should contain the following information for the technician:

1 A list and description of any modifications to be carried out to the waxed-up dentures or casts. It is advisable to have another trial insertion appointment after anything but the most minor modifications, and this is mandatory after re-recording the jaw relationship.

2 If the dentures are to be finished, the technician should be asked to add any wrought rests or clasps omitted from the trial insertion and to include palatal relief when indicated. The shade to be used for the pink acrylic resin should be specified. Any special finish (e.g. stippling) to be applied to the acrylic resin surface should be listed. A diagram of any stains to be incorporated into the pink resin or teeth must also be enclosed. If desired, the master cast should be duplicated so that the processed denture can be fitted on to the cast in the laboratory.

27 Insertion of the completed denture

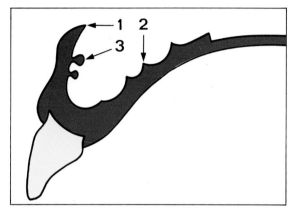

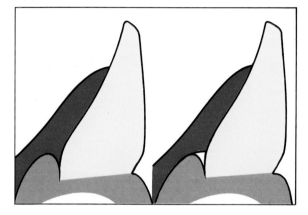

467 The denture is examined to ensure that the polished surfaces are well finished. The borders should be rounded and not sharp (1).

The impression surface should not have any sharp edges (2). These are commonly found in the area of the rugae and at the borders of a relief area. Any acrylic 'pearls' (3) should also be removed.

468 If acrylic resin has entered the gingival sulcus adjacent to the natural teeth (left), the resultant sharp ridge of acrylic should be eliminated (right). Care must be taken not to remove excess material, since the soft tissues are liable to proliferate into the space so created.

If the denture has been returned from the laboratory on duplicate casts, the latter should be examined for signs of abrasion produced by forcing rigid portions of the denture into place. Such abraded areas indicate parts of the denture which may require adjustment.

The denture is now seated in the mouth along the planned path of insertion and withdrawal. If it does not seat, it is likely to be due to acrylic having entered undercuts related to the natural teeth or the alveolar ridges. The area of acrylic involved may be detected by visual inspection or by the use of disclosing media as described in Chapter 24.

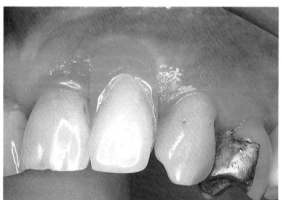

469 If the interference with insertion is related to a flange, the area responsible may be indicated by blanching of the mucosa as attempts are made to pass the acrylic flange over the most prominent part of the alveolar ridge.

470 The acrylic resin which hinders insertion of the denture (cross-hatched) is removed, taking care to preserve the contact between denture and hard and soft tissues in the non-undercut areas.

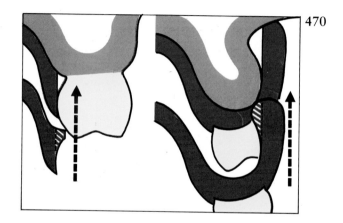

470

Once the denture is seated and is comfortable the fit of all its components is checked.

The denture should be retentive and stable. If free-end saddles rock about their most distal occlusal rests, this should be corrected by relining the saddles.

The occlusion is assessed from the patient's comments, visual inspection, articulating paper and shimstock.

471 Natural teeth may be separated by premature contacts on artificial teeth. The latter must be carefully adjusted until the natural teeth meet in precisely the same way with or without the denture in place. Where natural teeth do not indicate the desired jaw relationships, the artificial teeth must be adjusted to provide even occlusal contact at the optimal occlusal vertical dimension in the retruded jaw relationship. Further adjustment should be undertaken to permit even contact to be maintained in an intercuspal position slightly anterior to the retruded contact position.

In lateral and protrusive excursion the denture teeth should normally be adjusted so that they do not disturb the guidance offered by the remaining natural teeth.

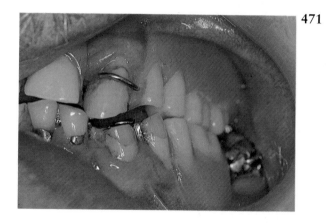

471

Articulating paper may help to localise any premature occlusal contact(s). The paper should be applied bilaterally in order to discourage deviation on closure of the mandible.

472 Heavy tooth contact is indicated by 'target' markings, having a light centre surrounded by a ring of ink transferred from the paper. Other marks, simply produced by the paper taking up the space between the teeth, are generally less distinct and lack the lighter centre. Differentiation between heavy and light tooth contacts can also be made with shimstock, which will easily pull out from between teeth not in firm contact.

The paper is relatively thick, and care must be taken to grind only those marks that indicate actual tooth contact.

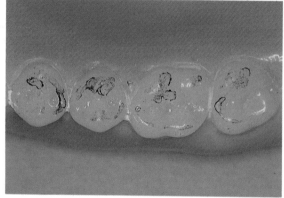

472

473

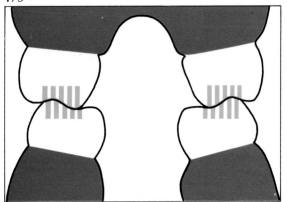

473 In those cases, where the partial denture saddles are extensive and the guidance in excursion from the remaining natural teeth allows the maintenance of bilateral balancing contacts, the following method of occlusal adjustment should be adopted. The occlusal vertical dimension is maintained by the upper palatal cusps and lower buccal cusps contacting the fossae of their opposing teeth. These are therefore known as *supporting* cusps.

474

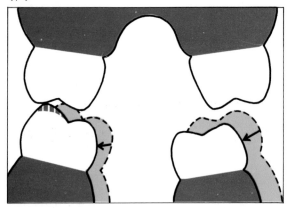

474 If one of these cusps contacts prematurely when the patient attempts to reach intercuspal position (blue) and is also premature in lateral excursions, the cusp is reduced in height.

475

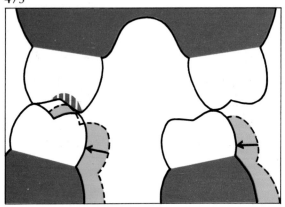

475 If the cusp contacts prematurely on closure as before, but is not premature in lateral excursions, the fossa is deepened.

Once even occlusal contact is achieved at the desired static jaw relationship, further adjustment of the supporting cusps should be avoided if possible.

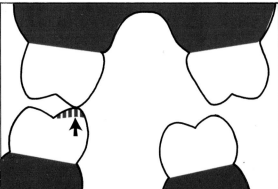

476 Thus if a premature contact occurs between a buccal upper cusp and a lower buccal cusp on the working side in lateral excursion, only the buccal upper (BU) cusp is adjusted.

477 Similarly, if in the same excursion, contact occurs between the upper palatal and lingual lower cusps, the lingual lower (LL) cusp is reduced. This method of adjusting tooth contact on the working side is thus called the BULL rule.

478 Premature contacts on the balancing side occur between supporting cusps. Such prematurities should be eliminated, wherever possible, by adjusting the area of interference rather than the area of support.

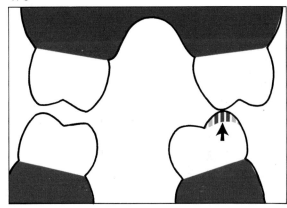

479 In protrusive excursion, premature contacts are eliminated by grinding the distal facing inclines of upper teeth and mesial facing inclines of lower teeth.

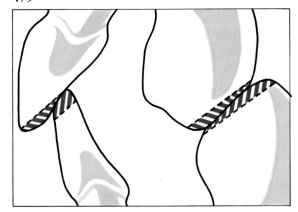

The patient is invited to check the appearance of the dentures so that any further minor modification can be carried out. After adjustments to the dentures have been completed, all areas that have been ground are repolished.

Instructions to the patient

Instructions to the patient should be given verbally and also reinforced with a printed sheet.

The explanation of any expected difficulties and limitations of the dentures made at the beginning of treatment should be reinforced. Despite the provision of retentive elements in the design, muscular control is very important in the successful wearing of dentures. Such control takes time to develop, so small quantities of non-sticky food should be chewed on both sides of the mouth initially.

The patient must be instructed in the correct path of insertion and removal of the dentures. Vulnerable components must be pointed out; thus clasps should not be used as finger-nail holds during removal.

480

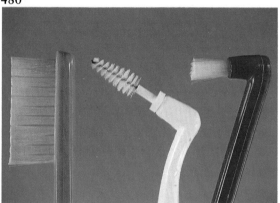

480 Detailed advice on denture hygiene should be provided. The patient should be encouraged to clean all surfaces of the dentures thoroughly after every meal. A small headed multitufted toothbrush has good access and adaptability to most of the surfaces; a single tufted (interspace) brush and/or a small bottle-type (interdental) brush may be required to clean the fitting surfaces of occlusal rests and clasps. Soap may be used on these brushes. However, some patients prefer to use toothpaste because of its flavour. In such cases, information on the brands which are least abrasive towards acrylic resin should be given.

The need for cleaning the remaining natural teeth should be stressed. Particular attention should be devoted to all surfaces covered by the denture. Patients should be asked to bring their toothbrush to the review appointment so that their brushing technique can be monitored and improved if required.

Disclosing solutions are useful aids for both patient and dentist to check the efficiency of cleansing of natural teeth and dentures.

To avoid fracture, dentures should be brushed over a basin half-full of water and they should not be squeezed in the palm of the hand.

Dentures should generally not be worn at night. However, patients may be advised to do so for the first week to aid adaptation. Immersion cleansers can be used as an adjunct to cleaning, but overnight soaking in the hypochlorite type may cause corrosion of cobalt chromium frameworks.

The patient should be advised that if significant discomfort is experienced during the first week the dentures should be removed and should not be worn again until a few hours before the review appointment. This short period of wear often aids the location of the cause of the pain.

The need for regular review of the mouth and denture should be emphasised. Not only may the natural teeth and periodontal tissues require treatment, but it is necessary to prevent damage from the denture which, in the initial stages, may be painless. For instance, free-end saddles may need to be relined in order to eliminate the rocking movement that could loosen abutment teeth and hasten loss of alveolar bone in the edentulous area. It must also be made clear that dentures have a limited life and therefore replacements will need to be constructed as appropriate.

The patient should be given an appointment for review in approximately seven days' time.

28 Review

Patients must be reviewed following the fitting of dentures to ensure that hard and soft tissues are not being damaged and that the dentures are functional. Any necessary denture adjustments are then carried out.

First review

The first review will usually be undertaken about one week after denture insertion. The patient is asked for comments on this initial period of denture wearing and a history is taken of any complaint. The most common complaints are of pain, or looseness, or both.

Even if the patient expresses complete satisfaction with the dentures, a careful examination of the mouth is essential. Because the patient may possess a high pain threshold or is reluctant to risk offending the dentist, evidence of damage caused by the denture may be found (even extensive ulceration) although the patient has reported that the dentures are entirely comfortable.

Information gleaned from the history of any complaint together with the findings on examination will guide the dentist to a diagnosis.

It is important to appreciate that discomfort and mucosal injury caused by the denture may be due either to faults relating to the impression surface or to the occlusal surface. It is easy to fall into the trap of concluding that mucosal damage in a particular instance is due to an error in the impression surface when this in fact is not the case, the danger being that ill-advised adjustment of that surface will almost certainly aggravate the situation.

Errors in the occlusion characteristically cause relatively diffuse mucosal damage. However, this is not always the case as other factors such as ridge morphology may serve to localise the effects of occlusal overload. For this reason, the occlusion must always be carefully assessed and the impression surface must never be adjusted empirically. Assessment of both the impression and occlusal surfaces will be made employing the procedures outlined in Chapters 24 and 27.

Impression surface faults

481 Since the ulcer in the left lower buccal sulcus is related to the denture border, the cause is most likely to be overextension. Where visibility is good the offending area of overextension can usually be easily identified and corrected. Visibility may be poor in the posterior region of the mouth and disclosing media may need to be used to ensure accurate location of the area of flange requiring adjustment.

481

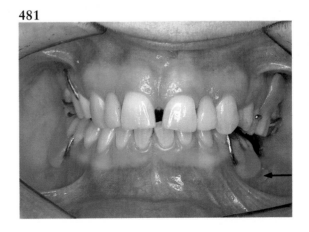

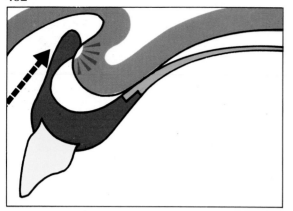

482 Ulceration of the most bulbous part of an undercut ridge is characteristic of inadequate relief of the undercut area resulting in trauma to the mucosa when the denture is inserted or removed.

The routine use of a disclosing agent to identify the area of impression surface involved is recommended.

Other causes of localised mucosal injury beneath the impression surface are acrylic pearls, or pressure points resulting from a damaged cast or inaccurate impression.

483

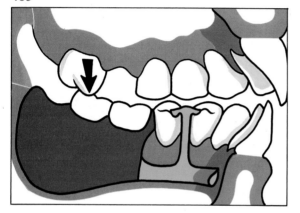

Occlusal surface faults

483 Lack of even contact in intercuspal position will load the supporting tissues unevenly as in this example of a free-end saddle denture with a premature contact in the second molar region.

Occlusal interference in lateral and protrusive excursions can displace the denture and thus traumatise the supporting tissues.

Occlusal errors can also cause facial discomfort and tenderness in the muscles of mastication as a result of the mandible manoeuvring to avoid the interferences.

Pain originating from the periodontal ligaments of teeth contacting the denture can arise from the application of excessive force either as the result of occlusal errors or inaccuracies in the fit of the denture. On rare occasions pulpal pain may result from galvanic action as a consequence of contact between a new metal framework and a freshly inserted amalgam restoration. The pain usually decreases with the passage of time as the surface of the amalgam tarnishes and the pulpal hyperaemia (consequent upon cavity preparation) subsides.

484

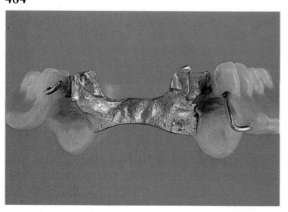

484 A reassessment of the patient's oral and denture hygiene forms an essential part of the review appointment. Disclosing solution (in this case blue) can be applied to teeth and dentures and the opportunity taken to reinforce the advice on plaque control already given. It may be necessary to modify the cleaning technique if the patient has obvious difficulty in removing plaque from certain areas. Any unevenness at the junction between acrylic and metal will also encourage plaque formation.

485

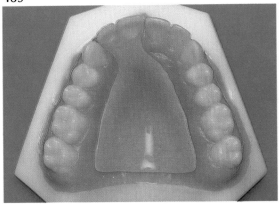

485 Dentures whose retention depends primarily on control by the patient's musculature may be reported as being loose if the patient has not yet developed the necessary skills. Further advice and encouragement may have to be given at this stage.

Subsequent reviews

If anything more than very minor tissue damage is noted at the first review an additional appointment may be required to ensure that healing has taken place.

If the patient is slow to acquire the neuro-muscular skills necessary for retention, it may be possible to modify the denture to increase physical retention.

Direct retention can sometimes be improved by adding a wrought clasp, and/or by modifying tooth contour by acid-etch composite additions (377).

Denture maintenance

Once problems arising directly after insertion of a denture have been resolved, regular inspection and maintenance of the denture is undertaken as part of the patient's routine dental care.

Unless there are regular inspections the denture can cause considerable damage which, at least in the early stages, may be symptomless; therefore the patient would not necessarily be aware that treatment is required. It is thus essential that when the dentures are fitted the need for regular recall appointments is emphasised to the patient.

Continued alveolar resorption, usually most marked under lower free-end saddles, progressively reduces mucosal support for dentures. When the effect of this on oral health and function is judged to be clinically significant a rebase to correct the lack of fit is indicated. The clinical procedure follows the principles laid down in Chapter 25.

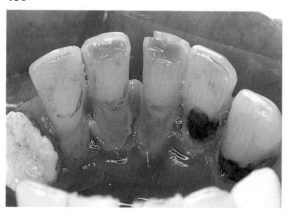

486 Failure to correct this deterioration at the appropriate time will result in damage to the tissues, such as mucosal inflammation, ulceration and hyperplasia, accelerated alveolar resorption and 'stripping' of the gingivae from the lingual aspects of the natural teeth, together with possibly increased tooth mobility.

487

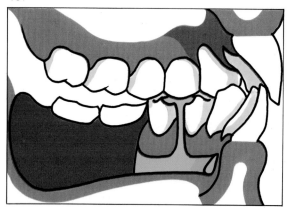

487 If alveolar resorption is accompanied by wear of the occlusal surface of the acrylic resin artificial teeth, the deranged occlusion will accelerate tissue damage. Simple rebasing of the saddles will not restore the correct occlusal contacts; the teeth can either be replaced or the dentures remade.

488

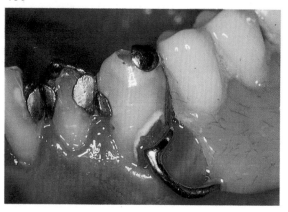

488 The routine oral review appointments are used to monitor the patient's level of plaque control and to reinforce this when necessary. Inadequate denture and oral hygiene can hasten the loss of natural teeth by caries and periodontal disease and may contribute to denture and angular stomatitis.

Maintenance may also, from time to time, involve repairs and additions to the dentures as described in Chapter 16.

Two contrasting clinical situations are offered at the end of this final chapter.

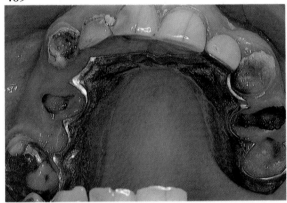

489

489 No one would deny that the long-term treatment of this patient has failed entirely.

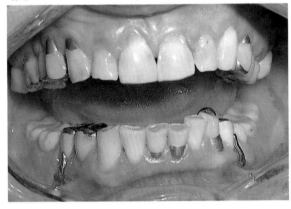

490

490 This patient has complemented the restorative treatment with a high standard of plaque control. There is no reason to doubt that the lower partial denture will continue to play a significant part in maintaining the health of the mouth as it has done in the previous four years.

Further reading

Textbooks and booklets

Basker R M, Harrison A and Ralph J P. Overdentures in general dental practice. London: British Dental Association, 1983.

Bates J F, Neill D J and Preiskel H W. Restoration of the Partially Dentate Mouth. Chicago: Quintessence, 1984.

Gross M D. Occlusion in Restorative Dentistry. Edinburgh: Churchill Livingstone, 1982.

Grundy J R. A Colour Atlas of Conservative Dentistry. London: Wolfe Medical Publications, 1980.

Henderson D and Steffel V L (ed). McCracken's Removable Partial Prosthodontics. 7th Ed. St. Louis: The C.V. Mosby Co, 1985.

Lammie G A and Laird W R E. Osborne and Lammie's Partial Dentures. 5th Ed. Oxford: Blackwell Scientific Publications, 1986.

Neill D J and Walter J D. Partial Denture Prosthetics. 2nd Ed. Oxford: Blackwell Scientific Publications, 1983.

Preiskel H W. Precision Attachments in Prosthodontics: The Application of Intracoronal and Extracoronal Attachments. Vol 1. Chicago: Quintessence, 1984.

Preiskel H W. Precision Attachments in Prosthodontics: Overdentures and Telescopic Prostheses. Vol 2. Chicago: Quintessence, 1985.

Pullen-Warner E and L'Estrange P R. Sectional Dentures, a Clinical and Technical Manual. Bristol: John Wright and Sons Ltd, 1978.

Strahan J D and Waite I M. A Colour Atlas of Periodontology. London: Wolfe Medical Publications, 1978.

Walter J D. Removable Partial Denture Design. London: British Dental Association, 1980.

Watt D M and MacGregor A R. Designing Partial Dentures. Bristol: Wright, 1984.

Wilson H J, Mansfield M A, Heath J R and Spence D. Dental Technology and Materials for Students. 8th Ed. Oxford: Blackwell Scientific Publications, 1987.

Zarb G A, Bergman B, Clayton J A and MacKay H F. Prosthodontic Treatment for Partially Edentulous Patients. St.Louis: The C.V. Mosby Co, 1978.

Zarb G A and Carlsson G E. Temporomandibular joint Function and Dysfunction. St.Louis: The C.V. Mosby Co, 1979.

Heintz W D (ed). Symposium on common failures in removable partial prosthodontics. The Dental Clinics of North America. 23, 1. Philadelphia: W.B. Saunders & Co, 1979.

Winkler S and Applebaum M (ed). Symposium on removable prosthodontics. The Dental Clinics of North America. 28, 2. Philadelphia: W.B. Saunders & Co, 1984.

Control of cross infection

British Dental Association: Guide to blood borne viruses and the control of cross infection in dentistry. London: 1987.

Dinsdale, R.C.W. Viral hepatitis, AIDS and dental treatment. British Dental Journal. London: 1985.

Design

Bracing and reciprocation

Kratochvil F J. Influence of occlusal rest position and clasp design on movement of abutment teeth. Journal of Prosthetic Dentistry 1963; *13:* 114–124.

Stern W J. Guiding planes in clasp reciprocation and retention. Journal of Prosthetic Dentistry 1975; *34:* 408–414.

Wiebelt F J and Stratton R J. Bracing and reciprocation in removable partial denture design. Quintessence of Dental Technology 1985; *9:* 15–17.

Connectors

Basker R M and Tryde G. Connectors for mandibular partial dentures: Use of the sublingual bar. Journal of Oral Rehabilitation 1977; *4:* 389–394.

Dyer M R Y. The acrylic lower partial denture. Dental Update 1984; *11:* 401-410.

Reitz P V and Caputo A A. A photoelastic study of stress distribution by a mandibular split major connector. Journal of Prosthetic Dentistry 1985; *54:* 220–225.

Design prescription

Basker R M and Davenport J C. A survey of partial denture design in general dental practice. Journal of Oral Rehabilitation 1978; *5:* 215–222.

Miller E L. Systems for classifying partially edentulous arches. Journal of Prosthetic Dentistry 1970; *24:* 25–40.

Schwarz W D and Barsby M J. Design of partial dentures in dental practice. Journal of Dentistry 1978; *2:* 166–170.

Retention

Basker R M. Clinical evaluation of partial denture retainers. *In* Bates J F, Neill D J and Preiskel H W (ed). Restoration of the Partially Dentate Mouth, pp. 211–223. Chicago: Quintessence, 1984.

Bates J F. Retention of partial dentures. British Dental Journal 1980; *149:* 171–174.

Browning J D, Jameson W L, Stewart C D, McGarrah H E and Eick J D. Effect of positional loading of three removable partial denture clasp assemblies on movement of abutment teeth. Journal of Prosthetic Dentistry 1986; *55:* 347–351.

Cunningham J L. Clasping using Wiptam wrought wire. Journal of Dentistry 1985; *13:* 311–317.

Demer W J. An analysis of mesial rest-I-bar clasp designs. Journal of Prosthetic Dentistry 1976; *36:* 243–253.

Frank R P, Brudvik J S and Nicholls J I. A comparison of the flexibility of wrought wire and cast circumferential clasps. Journal of Prosthetic Dentistry 1983; *49:* 471–476.

Hebel K S, Graser G N and Featherstone J D B. Abrasion of enamel and composite resin by removable partial denture clasps. Journal of Prosthetic Dentistry 1984; *52:* 389–397.

Kratochvil F J and Caputo A A. Photoelastic analysis of pressure on teeth and bone supporting removable partial dentures. Journal of Prosthetic Dentistry 1974; *32:* 52–61.

Krol A J. RPI (Rest, Proximal Plate, I Bar). Clasp retainer and its modifications. Dental Clinics of North America 1973; *17:* 631–649.

Matheson G R, Brudvik J S and Nicholls J I. Behaviour of wrought wire clasps after repeated permanent deformation. Journal of Prosthetic Dentistry 1986; *55:* 226–231.

Morris H F, Ajgar K, Brudvik J S, Winkler S and Roberts E P. Stress relaxation testing. Part IV: Clasp pattern dimensions and their influence on clasp behaviour. Journal of Prosthetic Dentistry 1983; *50:* 319–326.

Ralph J P. Laboratory assessment of the influence of clasp design on the abutment teeth and supporting tissues. *In* Bates J F, Neill D J and Preiskel H W (ed). Restoration of the Partially Dentate Mouth, pp. 203–209. Chicago: Quintessence, 1984.

Simmons J J. The role of swing-lock partial dentures. *In* Bates J F, Neill D J and Preiskel H W (ed). Restoration of the Partially Dentate Mouth, pp. 299–308. Chicago: Quintessence, 1984.

Wright S M. The use of spring-loaded attachments for retention of removable partial dentures. Journal of Prosthetic Dentistry 1984; *51:* 605–610.

Support

Becker C M and Kaldahl W B. Support for the distal extension removable partial denture. International Journal of Periodontics and Restorative Dentistry 1983; *3:* 29–37.

Fisher R L. Factors that influence the base stability of mandibular distal-extension removable partial dentures: A longitudinal study. Journal of Prosthetic Dentistry 1983; *50:* 167–171.

Manderson R D. The role of tooth and mucosal support in prosthodontics. *In* Bates J F, Neill D J and Preiskel H W (ed). Restoration of the Partially Dentate Mouth, pp. 237–245. Chicago: Quintessence, 1984.

Watt D M, MacGregor A R, Geddes M, Cockburn A and Boyd J L. A preliminary investigation of the support of partial dentures and its relationship to occlusal loads. Dental Practitioner 1958; *9:* 2–15.

Jaw relationships and occlusion

Brill N and Tryde G. Physiology of mandibular positions. Frontiers of Oral Physiology 1974; *1:* 199–237.

Pietrokovski J and Neill D J. Occlusion in the partially dentate mouth. *In* Bates J F, Neill D J and Preiskel H W (ed). Restoration of the Partially Dentate Mouth pp. 273–283. Chicago: Quintessence 1984.

Winstanley R. The hinge axis – a review of the literature. Journal of Oral Rehabilitation 1985; *21:* 135–159.

Zarb G A and Mackay H F. The occlusal surface in removable partial prosthodontics. *In* Lundeen H C and Gibbs C C (ed). Advances in Occlusion. Postgraduate Dental Handbook Series, Vol. *14* pp. 161–167. Bristol: John Wright, 1982.

Partial dentures and oral health

Abelson D C. Denture plaque and denture cleansers: a review of the literature. Gerodontics 1985; *5:* 202–206.

Augsburger R H and Elahi J M. Evaluation of seven proprietary denture cleansers. Journal of Prosthetic Dentistry 1982; *47:* 356–359.

Bates J F. Plaque accumulation and partial denture design. *In* Bates J F, Neill D J and Preiskel H W (ed). Restoration of the Partially Dentate Mouth. pp. 225–236. Chicago: Quintessence, 1984.

Berg E. Periodontal problems associated with use of distal extension removable partial dentures – a matter of construction? Journal of Oral Rehabilitation 1985; *12:* 369–379.

Budtz-Jorgenson E. Oral mucosal lesions associated with the wearing of removable dentures. Journal of Oral Pathology 1981; *10:* 65–80.

Carlsson G E, Hedegård B and Koivumaa K K. Studies in partial denture prosthesis IV. Final results of a 4-year longitudinal investigation of dentogingivally supported partial dentures. Acta Odontologica Scandinavica 1965; *23:* 443–472.

Chandler J A and Brudvik J S. Clinical evaluation of patients eight to nine years after placement of removable partial dentures. Journal of Prosthetic Dentistry 1984; *51:* 736–743.

Germundsson B, Hellman M and Odman P. Effects of rehabilitation with conventional removable partial dentures. Swedish Dental Journal 1984; *8:* 171–182.

Gunne H-S J. The effect of removable partial dentures on mastication and dietary intake. Acta Odontologica Scandinavica 1985; *43:* 269–278.

Koivumaa K K, Anderson J N and Hedegård B. Some aspects of partial dentures. International Dental Journal 1959; *9:* 30–40.

Osborne J, Brill N and Hedegård B. The nature of prosthetic dentistry. International Dental Journal 1966; *16:* 509–526.

Wagg B J. Root surface caries: A review. Community Dental Health 1984; *1:* 11–20.

Tooth preparation

Schwarz W D and Barsby M J. Tooth alteration procedures prior to partial denture construction, Parts 1–3. Dental Update 1984; *11:* 19–34, 167–178, 231–237.

Smith B J. Abutment preparation for removable partial dentures. *In* Bates J F, Neill D J and Preiskel H W (ed). Restoration of the Partially Dentate Mouth, pp. 259–271. Chicago: Quintessence, 1984.

Watson R M. Guide planes. *In* Bates J F, Neill D J and Preiskel H W (ed). Restoration of the Partially Dentate Mouth, pp. 193–201. Chicago: Quintessence, 1984.

Terminology and standards

Academy of Denture Prosthetics: Glossary of prosthodontic terms, edited by the Nomenclature Committee, ed. 4, St.Louis: The C.V. Mosby Co, 1977.

British Society for the Study of Prosthetic Dentistry. Guides to Standards in Prosthetic Dentistry. British Dental Journal 1981; *150:* 167–169.

British Standards Glossary of Dental Terms, BS4492. London: British Standards Institution, 1983.

Index

Numbers in light type refer to pages; those in **bold** type refer to illustrations.